ALSO BY JIM COOPER
TWISTED TIES

The (Not So) Little Book of Cancer Caregiving

>>>>>>>>>>>>>>>>>>>>>>>>>>>>>>>>

How To Be A
CAREGIVER WARRIOR
and Keep Your Sanity

>>>>>>>>>>>>>>>>>>>>>>>>>>>>>>>>

Jim Cooper

FACEPLANT BOOKS LLC   DELAWARE

JIM COOPER

Copyright © 2023 by Jim Cooper/FacePlant Books LLC
All rights reserved.

No part of this book may be reproduced by any mechanical, photographic, or electronic process, or in the form of an audio recording; nor may it be stored in a retrieval system, transmitted, or otherwise be copied for public or private use - other than for "fair use" as brief quotations embodied in articles and reviews - without prior written permission of the publisher.

The author of this book does not dispense medical advice or other professional advice or prescribe the use of any technique as a form of diagnosis or treatment for any physical, emotional, or medical condition. The intent of the author is only to offer information of an anecdotal and general nature that may be part of your quest for emotional and spiritual well-being. In the event you or others use any information or other content in this book, the author and the publisher assume no responsibility for the direct or indirect consequences. The reader should consult his or her medical, health, or other professional before adopting any of the suggestions in this book or drawing inferences from it. For further information contact:

FacePlant Books LLC
216 Sundance Ln
Milton, DE 19968

ISBN: 978-0-9888213-2-3

1st Trade Paperback Edition, July 2023

Cover Design, Print Design & Dancing Frogs Trained by: Jim Cooper
100% Human hand-crafted. No AI Tools were used to create text or any graphical element of this work.

For Sally.
Not many women would undergo cancer treatment just to provide a book-worthy subject for their ersatz author lesser half. You are the model of courage and fortitude. How could I not love you?

To the Memory of Steve Baldwin.
Husband, Father, Singer, Musician, Fighter. Cancer won this round, but you left us the courage to continue the war.

To the Memory of Rose & Pete Milazzo.
Together forever.

The Tips & Other Stuff

Introduction — 1
    So what scares the hell out of you?

Caregiver Tip # 1 — 5
    Being scared to death is normal. Breathe.

Caregiver Tip # 2 — 19
    Denial is common for caregivers and families.
    Don't fight it; work with it

Caregiver Tip # 3 — 31
    Stop looking up everything on the Internet.

Caregiver Tip # 4 — 37
    Adjust your life to allow space for cancer.

Caregiver Tip # 5 — 49
    Maintain an Attitude of Gratitude.
    Things could be worse.

Caregiver Tip # 6 — 67
    Trust your instincts.
    Tune into the gentle voice in your head
    It will guide you where you need to go

Caregiver Tip # 7 — 79
    Spirituality. Get some.

Caregiver Tip # 8 — 95
    You are not alone. Caregiving is a team sport. Take advantage of everyone who comes into your inner circle.

Caregiver Tip # 9 — 123
    Make self-care a priority. Pay attention to your own needs.

Caregiver Tip # 10 — 133
    Get organized.

Caregiver Tip # 11 — 147
    Holidays will be different. Plan ahead.

Caregiver Tip # 12 — 163
    Find distractions to minimize the constant medical focus, for the patient and yourself.

Caregiver Tip # 13 — 173
    Celebrate everything. No matter how small.

Caregiver Tip # 14 — 183
 Doctors are the mechanics. Nurses are the healers.
 Treat them as such.

Caregiver Tip # 15 — 195
 Be flexible.
 Allow for sudden unexpected shifts in the process.
 They will happen.

Caregiver Tip # 16 — 205
 Bad days happen.
 Remember they don't last forever.
 Focus on taking one step at a time and trust tomorrow will be better.

Caregiver Tip # 17 — 225
 Help other caregivers.
 Listen.
 Share your experience.

Caregiver Tip # 18 — 233
 Don't shy away from conversations about death and dying.

Caregiver Tip # 19 — 243
 Don't shy away from conversations about money and finances.

Caregiver Tip # 20 — 249
 Give yourself credit. Learn to accept praise from others.

Caregiver Tip # 21 — 259
 I'm sure you've noticed that everything has changed.
 Go easy on yourself while you adjust to the hew norm.

Caregiver Tip # 22 — 267
 As treatment wanes, take the time to decompress.
 It's okay, and sometimes necessary, to seek outside help.

Post Script — 275

Caregiver Warriors — 279
 Thank you. Thank you. Thank you. Thank you.

Appendix A: Caregiver Resources — 283

Appendix B: Signs of Caregiver Burnout — 285

Appendix C: Financial Resources — 286

Bibliography — 289

About the Author — 291

So.... What Scares the Hell Out of You???

Introduction

Insects? SNAKES? Flying (guilty)? **Bridges?** FIRE, BATS, TSUNAMI, The Boogeyman?

Pfft. Child's play.

Try this on for size...

YOU HAVE CANCER

When I first heard those words uttered in the direction of Sally, my wife, every nerve in my body exploded, I went stone cold deaf and felt the earth stand still. Okay, maybe not that last one but absolutely the first two.

What you are now reading is how I, as a reluctant volunteer to the ranks of caregiving, forged ahead, through the fear and into a world I never knew existed. Along the way I witnessed courage, empathy, sadness, panic, grief, love, joy and a connection with more glorious people than I ever thought possible.

HOWEVER — The biggest lesson I learned? Caregiving is not a walk in the park. The health care industry is beginning to come to grips with the stress and consequences caregivers face. This book is my two cents of what I experienced, the good and the bad, and some general guidelines that made the trip bearable, and at times wonderful. My wish is that it gives you a head start on your journey and provides at least a modicum of reassurance that you are not alone - and help is always available.

What follows are basic guidelines to caregiver self-care; ones that I experienced first hand and have since been reinforced by many caregiver resources - most of which are listed in the back of this book. With each guideline, I shared part of our journey through the world of cancer. The book is structured so you can skip all that if you want and just focus on the guidelines. They are worth referring to repeatedly - I know I had to remind myself of them often. I hope my words bring you a tiny bit of peace and comfort.

> *"All I ever wanted since I arrived here on Earth were the things that turned out to be within reach. The same things I needed as a baby - to go from cold to warm, lonely to held, the vessel to the giver, empty to full. You can change the world with a hot bath, if you sink into it from a place of knowing that you are worth profound care, even when you're dirty and rattled.*
> *Who knew?"*
> *~ Anne Lamott*

Being scared to death...is normal. Breathe.

Caregiver Tip #1

The hardest and scariest part of the journey is the seemingly endless time spent "not knowing." Downtime between appointments or waiting for test results to return, found me sitting around with a continuous loop of doomsday scenarios flashing through my brain. At the start I didn't even know what questions to ask. All I knew was that something was wrong...and I wanted answers. Those answers took awhile. It's normal to be scared to death while waiting for those answers. Remembering to breathe helps.

Caregiver quote: "Remember to take a few deep breaths every day. Just that small act would slow down my racing heart and clear my mind. I wish had known to do this right from the beginning of my son's journey."

In The Beginning...

Breaking down the bathroom door of a complete stranger's beach house was not on my to-do list on a hot Saturday in July, but that's what I was forced to do. Bill's wife Mary had looked at me with pained eyes, pointed to the bathroom, and asked me in her light Scottish accent, "Is Sally okay? I think she might need your help."

She was right, but I already knew that. I saw it coming a hundred miles away.

We were attending a reunion of sorts; my college mates Bill, Keith, Dave and Rich had arranged a little get together at a house on Long Beach Island that Dave and his wife Sue were renting for the week. On the drive there, I was a kid on Christmas Eve, excitement and anticipation pumping obscene levels of adrenaline into my system. During college these people were my family. True we had not seen each other often since graduation, but I had forged bonds fused with crazy glue - time and distance meant zero.

Upon arrival the tableau was staged as expected, everyone gathered with some sort of alcoholic concoction in-hand. Rich, naturally, manned the blender, whipping up lethal drinks for which the device has yet to be invented that could measure the alcohol content.[1]

---

[1] Rich's idea of a Manhattan was three ice cubes, two dashes of bitters, one day-glo maraschino cherry and a Big Gulp amount of bourbon. Skoal.

In order to record the occasion before anyone lost the ability to walk a straight line, we tromped to the beach so we could take photos to confirm who still had their hair (Keith), and who was still in shape (Keith - bastard).

Sally and the beach are one. It's her favorite happy place where she totally relaxes. On our beach vacations, she's ensconced in the sand by nine in the morning and aside from lunch and bathroom breaks, she remains there until mid-afternoon. It is the only place where she's able to let everything go.

After the pictures were taken, Sally and I stood in the sand watching the waves crash on shore. The on-shore breeze tousled Sally's short brown hair, her dark eyes focused on the ocean, drinking in what little serenity could be grabbed. Sally wore her emotions on her face. As she stood, feet buried in the sand, wearing jeans and a white peasant top, I could tell she pictured herself in a swimsuit and beach chair, letting the sun massage her soul into tranquility.

"We'll get back here next year," I said. We had put off our beach trip that season. During the summer of 2014, our time, and a large chunk of our disposable cash, was allocated to selling the townhouse that was our home for almost 30 years and moving to new digs.

"I know," she said. "Just not doable right now."

We all walked back to the house talking, laughing and still catching up with each other's lives. Nothing was out of the ordinary.

Not more than five minutes later, Sally and I were parked on the living room sofa, and it dawned on me that that she had suddenly grown unusually quiet. One look at her told me why.

Sally's eyes were thoroughly glazed over and not focused on much of anything. I'd seen that face before. The drinks had done their job: She was thoroughly trashed and was going to be sick.

I was dumbfounded. She'd instantly gone from coherent and jovial to a condition reminiscent of alcohol poisoning. It did not dawn on me at that time how fast this had happened; if it had, perhaps my reaction would have been more sympathetic and less petulant. Instead, immediately and selfishly, I was royally pissed off. How could she pull this shit knowing how important this party was to me? A distant sense of dread rose in my gut, but I pushed it aside in hopes that ignoring what was happening was the best solution.

Willing the most even-tempered voice I could muster I asked, "Are you okay?"

"I'm fine," she slurred.[2]

I sensed everyone else was beginning to suspect something was amiss. Keith asked Sally a direct question about her recent job and, after she made a few gulping sounds, I quickly answered for her and steered the conversation elsewhere. My guts tightened a few more notches as it became more and more apparent that this was not going to end well.

After Mary's comment, I put my weight to the bathroom door as Sally was making a feeble attempt to block it, not knowing who was trying to enter. I was surprised she could muster any rational thought.

Bursting through the door, she was somehow still on her feet, bent at the waist over the sink, eyes shut, pants around her ankles.

"Are you okay?" I asked, not being able to think of anything else to say. Sally gurgled a few incoherent sounds in response as I sat her back on the toilet just to keep her from falling and hurting herself; I wasn't entirely sure that had not happened already. Her body had let loose from every possible

---

2   "I'm fine", in Sally's case, is code for Sound Red Alert. Strap in, get the crew to their battle stations, and go to DEFCON 1. The "I'm fine" beast would rear its gruesome head repeatedly over the next couple years, always signaling a torpedo in the water.

orifice; her shirt vomit stained. Fortunately, she was sitting on the john when all systems let loose.

I had to get her out of there, but I really didn't want to walk her out in puke drenched clothing. Stuffing all my humiliation as deeply as possible, I left Sally sitting, completely bent over at the waist, granted a stupid move as it was the perfect position for a head-first swan dive into the tile floor.

Coming out of the bathroom, my guts twisted a bit more as all eyes fell on me questioning what the hell was going on.

"Can I borrow a t-shirt or something from someone, please?" I said.

Dave produced one of his, which was perfect considering his six-foot plus frame. I changed Sally, cleaned up the bathroom, got her on her feet - or at least held her up to look like she was on her feet - and we made our way straight to our car. I don't remember if I said good-bye to anyone. I didn't have the courage to look anyone in the eye, thinking the embarrassment would kill me.

Keith followed us out to make sure we were all right. He said, "We love you, Sally" as I poured her into the backseat in the prone position, passed out cold.

On the drive home through the New Jersey Pine Barrens, I was busy feeling sorry for myself and growing angrier by the mile. I was thoroughly humiliated in front of the people who meant the most to me during our four-year stint at college. What I had built up in my mind as the best time I would have, probably for all of 2014, crashed and burned because my wife decided to get completely shit-faced. I entertained pulling the car over and tossing Sally into the woods and leaving her there. She would never know the difference until possibly the next day. By then I could have moved to Florida, or Canada, where starting a new life was a huge possibility.

Once home I guided Sally into bed, put the garbage can on the floor next to her, just in case, sent a quick email of apology to the crew, and tried to breathe normally. Like Fred Flintstone, my conscience appeared in the form of two tiny figures, a white haloed angel on one shoulder and the pitchforked devil on the other. War waged between my ears, the skirmish determining where I would land, homicide or forgiveness. Interlaced with the emotional turmoil was the logical side trying to figure out what the fuck had just happened. I've seen Sally smashed before, but this was different. I held the garbage can for her after a particularly raucous New Year's Eve, but she had never dropped into incoherence, lost the ability to communicate, or lost control over bodily functions.

I needed to chill and needed to let go of all the self-destructive thoughts buzzing in my head; I sought refuge on our back patio. The tops of the trees in the backyard were on fire with the hot July sunset; the leaves danced in the dragon's breath of a breeze. I focused on just trying to breathe, practicing all the Zen awareness that therapy had pounded into me. The bottom line, once I got past all the bluster and anger keeping me protected, was that I was scared. Big time.

As I sat watching the day move from the orange of sunset to the purple of evening, the afternoon's events looped repeatedly through my head, not so much to relive the embarrassment, but looking for some hint, some clue as to what had happened. An allergic reaction of some kind? Alcohol poisoning? The unnerving thought that she had suffered some sort of stroke kept rearing its ugly face.

Sally remained comatose until the next morning, but upon awakening remained sick as two dogs.

"I am so sorry," she said, white faced and ashamed. "I don't know what happened."

"How many drinks did you have?" I asked, giving her a hug. Obviously the white-haloed shoulder guy won - game, set, and match.

"Just one," she said, the memory of which turned her face nauseatingly green.

I put her back under the covers, surprised that 15 hours later she was still physically ill, especially if her memory of ingesting only one drink was accurate. Perhaps she was dealing with some sort of food poisoning. No single explanation seemed to explain all of Sally's symptoms and reactions, although in my mind, stroke was still the leading contender.

Over the next few days my feelings of humiliation and anger dissipated. The world didn't end, and life's routine resumed. At least for a little while….

A week later I was home when Sally returned from her job as admin at a small social services office. I could see she was visibly upset, glassy eyed and her face sagged with disappointment and worry.

"What's going on?" I asked.

In stuttering sentences she said, "That office is crazy. I can't do everything they want me to do."

"Such as?"

She dumped her purse on the chair and slumped into the couch in the den. "I've got to answer the phones, deal with the insurance companies, and all the doctors are constantly buzzing me with requests for this patient and that, setting up their medications and getting their next appointments set."

Outwardly I was being sympathetic but inwardly I didn't see the issue. For someone who thrived on being busy, this didn't sound like anything she had not come across in any previous job. She had once been an executive administrator for a bigwig at Merrill Lynch without breaking a sweat. She ran a social services office three times the size of her current job and never had a problem with the workload. It didn't make any sense to me that this small counseling office could be so overwhelming. In the far-reaches of my mind, nasty little fear-microbs were trying to nudge me into connecting recent events, the word "stroke" reappeared, but I quickly repressed it in hopes of holding on to life as we knew it.

Four days out of five, Sally would return home in the same state of frustration. My solution, which required little thought, was just to quit. That's not Sally's nature; she hangs on to her commitments, sometimes past the point of her own mental health.

Saturday provided a bit of breathing space for both of us. I was out running errands when I sent Sally a text message:

"You want me to pick up a sandwich at Wawa for you?"

The response, which took an unusual amount of time to arrive, was

"Th wr5tg goode."

Several succeeding texts from Sally showed the same tendencies to make little or no sense. Even so, this was one more thing I conveniently ignored for the sake of maintaining normalcy.

One aspect to which I could no longer shut my eyes was the deterioration of Sally's motor skills. In addition to an increasing number of drinking glasses that she failed to maintain a grasp upon, and consequently smashing on the floor, Sally's arms had taken on a life of their own. Reaching for a teacup, her arm would get halfway there and detour out into space for a few seconds before reaching its target. It looked as if she was standing on the tarmac of a major airport flagging in 747s.

In late August, we went out to dinner at a new restaurant that was somewhere between casual and fine dining, sporting fancy wine glasses and white linen tablecloths, but still featured basic American fare. Every two minutes a loud clang echoed throughout the restaurant as a knife or fork fell out of Sally's hand and slammed onto the plate. My self-consciousness kicked into red alert, and I held my breath every time she picked up a drinking glass, waiting for it to crash to the floor.

I don't know why this was the moment where it all came together; when everything that had happened in the past two months coalesced in my brain as a series of connected events: getting blackout drunk, the text messages, the job, the arm movements. A calm sense of realization broke through all my defenses; not in a burst of anger or craziness, but in a gentle knowing that the time to act had arrived.

"It's time to go see the doctor," I said.

To my surprise, Sally said, "Okay." I expected reluctance on Sally's part, so I felt a huge sense of relief at her agreement. I was still not convinced that my stroke theory was wrong as her errant behaviors had become more frequent. Even more frightening, Sally was still behind the wheel of a car.

The night prior to our scheduled appointment with the doctor, we were in the kitchen cleaning up after dinner, Sally rinsing dishes and utensils and me loading them in the dishwasher. She handed me a dinner plate and said, "Here. Put this in the laundry."

I grabbed the plate and stopped cold. "Excuse me?" I said.

"Yeah, in the laundry," Sally said continuing to rinse the flatware, as if nothing were amiss.

The following morning she held a drinking glass in her hand and stated, "I really like this car."

I was on the verge of quietly freaking out.

The next day we visited Dr. Lou Tsarouhas, our family doctor since the early 1990's. Well loved and respected, over the years, we had established a trusting relationship with Lou.[3] We explained to him what was going on and that the onset of this appeared to be the alcohol reaction at the party.

He put Sally through a battery of motion tests, making her walk heel to toe, holding her arms out straight, touching her finger to her nose with her eyes closed. He concluded, "It's not a stroke." I felt the tension flood out of my body, but that was short lived.

He said, "I want you to see a neurologist, and he'll probably want you to get an MRI."

An MRI? Seriously? I thought, can't we just clear this up with some Bactine and a couple Tylenol?

---

[3] Except when he bitched at me about my weight. In that aspect I felt his philosophy was to the extreme right of Lester Maddox.

Here's what's scaring me right now:

_____
_____
_____
_____
_____
_____
_____
_____
_____
_____
_____

The action I will take is:

_____
_____
_____
_____
_____
_____
_____

Notes:

Caregiver Tip #2

Denial is common for caregivers and families. Don't fight it; work with it.

Denial is not necessarily a bad thing. It's a form of self-protection, especially in the face of terrifying circumstances. It can, however, become a roadblock for caregivers and patients alike. Talk to people - family, friends, professionals. Share what you know to get different perspectives.

A big clue that denial is becoming too powerful? How easily does anger rise to the surface?

Skyscraper-sized murals of Big Bird, Elmo and Oscar the Grouch ushered us to the office of Dr. Steven Mazlin, the neurologist destined to peek at Sally's brain. His office was accessible primarily through the main entrance to Sesame Place, a popular Sesame Street-based amusement park in eastern Pennsylvania. The road to Dr. Mazlin's office bisected the amusement park parking lot. Bert and Ernie's play area and was equipped with a stop light at the midway point to control pedestrian traffic. It's easy to tell which direction the parents and kids were headed; it's all in the parents' faces. Heading into the park, Mom and Dad were alert and in command, trying to maintain control of excited children. Those heading back to their SUVs pushed strollers overloaded with comatose children buried under overpriced Sesame Place plush toys and plastic junk, the parents' faces a weary, drawn mask as if suffering from a novocaine overdose.

Dr. Mazlin was a soft-spoken young man with an openly gentle and round face, and his eyes radiated an uncanny intelligence. Decorating the walls of his office were newspaper clippings not highlighting his medical achievements, but the successes he had with his primary hobby, astrophotography, accompanied by photographic glimpses of the heavens he'd taken from various observatories. I could see why neurology fascinated him. The semi-opaque brain lesions that appeared in MRI pictures were not unlike the far-distant star clusters and supernovas.

Such were the results of Sally's MRI Dr. Mazlin displayed for us on his computer, dozens of white clouds floating in all directions, most of them small and semi-transparent, but there was one that was a bit larger and less opaque than the others.

"If the MRI showed just this one bigger spot," Dr. Mazlin explained, "I'd say we were talking about a tumor. But with all these other lesions, I think it's more along the lines of MS."

Not great news but better than a tumor for God's sake. At this point I would have been okay with amputation as long as I could keep "cancer" tucked safely away in a dark recess where an unimaginable fear lurked.

Dr. Mazlin continued, "If it is MS, it is very treatable with the drugs that have been developed. This could also be a one-time event. It's possible to treat these lesions, and they may disappear and not return."

So we learned another new vocabulary word, ADEM, which is infinitely easier to say than Acute Disseminated Encephalomyelitis. In normal-speak, it means a brief, one-time inflammation of the brain and/or spinal cord. This was Dr. Mazlin's possible one-time event. I was mentally betting the farm on ADEM, getting quickly past this, and moving on with our lives.

"The first thing we are going to do," he continued, "is blast these lesions with steroids."

"When?" I asked.

"Now."

Now? Friday at four in the afternoon? Registering the urgency of what was happening was not a place I wanted to go. That, in itself, cranked the fear level up a notch.

The plan of attack was three, successive days of high-dose steroid infusion followed by a week of oral steroids in hopes of eliminating, or at the least, reducing the size of the all the lesions on Sally's brain. Luckily, the infusion could take place at our local hospital, the Princeton Medical

Center, a facility that had recently moved from downtown Princeton to a new glass and chrome building in Plainsboro.

On the way to the hospital, Sally said, "We have to…" Silence.

"Have to…?" I asked.

An empty concentration filled her eyes. This had become familiar territory, and from here it was a guessing game to determine what her original thought contained.

I said, "Have to…go?"

She shook her head.

"Have to…pick up something?"

"No," she mumbled staring straight ahead, staring into emptiness devoid of the ability to think.

"Have to…call someone?"

Frustration appeared on her face, and she shook her head, "No. Forget it."

Sometimes I guessed a word that kick-started her brain, and she was able to complete her thought. Sometimes not. Sally's ability to communicate came and went without any logical pattern. I could not imagine the frustration of being unable to think and articulate a need or desire, existing as a fifty-eight-year-old with a constantly short-circuiting mental capacity.

Depending on the source, the word "hospital" derives from either the Latin hospes or the Latin hospitale, both of which are also the recorded roots of the words hospitiable, hospice, hotel…hostage. That was certainly accurate.

As we entered the emergency area of Princeton Medical Center, I felt as if we were making the prisoner's march across the Bridge of Sighs. The room was institutionally lit and featured waiting area furniture covered in washable vinyl the color of Pepto-Bismol.

"Sally Cooper," I said to the cherubic ER attendant, a young lady who smiled in the face of all incoming diseases, complaints and open wounds, even at four on a Friday afternoon. "She is supposed to get a steroid infusion."

A few keyboard clicks and she said, "Oh, yes. Mrs. Cooper. Let me tell them you are here." They were waiting for us.

Not two minutes later a dark-skinned woman dressed in medical blues sauntered through the doors that lead back to the guts of the ER. "Mrs. Cooper," she said, her smiling West Indian accent immediately cut through the tension I felt. "How are you, my dear?"

Sally smiled weakly. "If I was good, I wouldn't be here."

"Come with me, then. We'll get you fixed up." Her smile never left her face.

We were lead through a labyrinth of hallways into a large room that reminded me of a church basement recreation area filled with cubicles constructed in rows like any good corporate office. Each cube had an oversized, olive green, La-Z-Boy chair and a small flat screen TV on a wall-mounted swivel arm. Most man-caves aren't that well-appointed.

"Mrs. Cooper, do you have a port? No? That's okay. I will put a pic line in your arm and get you hooked up to the IV."

"How long will the..." Sally lost the words but made a pointing motion in the air to the empty IV stand.

"How long will the drip take?" the nurse asked and Sally nodded. "It should take about 90 minutes."

With the drip underway, the nurse said, "If you need anything, Sally, you just let me know." They had moved onto a first-name basis. The room had a chill in the air so even though it was warm and humid outside,

Sally was snuggled into the chair under a couple hospital blankets and was starting to doze in front of the TV screen.

My responsibilities at this point were to watch. That got old after about five minutes.

I realized official communication responsibilities to family and friends was now in my domain. Sally's ancient Egyptian, hieroglyphic text messages were not going to cut it. Broaching the topic of relinquishing her phone to me was only slightly less painful than sequestering her kids, grandkids and siblings in undisclosed locations.

Some families are close, some not so much. Sally's biological family members are all hard-wired to each other, which is a good thing most of the time, but sometimes can be a complete pain in the ass when opinions differ.[1]

In crisis situations such as this, however, no one rallies faster than Sally's siblings and relatives, they supported each other in any way possible. I had a feeling Sally's sister Katie was going to ride shotgun with me throughout whatever was coming. She was closest geographically and emotionally, living 15 minutes from our house and having been, more or less, raised by her older sister.

Consequently, our own kids, Stephen and Beth, were cut from the same cloth, and aside from being angry and scared that their Mother had to deal with more than a minor medical issue, they would jump at the chance to do whatever needed to be done.

Sally's support network beyond family was extensive; I was looking at a full-time job trying to keep everyone informed. Thankfully, we live in the age of electronic communications; otherwise I'd have to spend my days with my phone crazy-glued to my head.

---

[1] Imagine Gordon Ramsey, Michael Irvine, Anne Burrell, and Jacques Pepin all cooking the same dish at the same time. In a single pot.

I took advantage of the downtime during infusion to compose the first family broadcast email:

To:
From:
Subject: Sally Status

All-

Sally has several areas of inflammation in her brain. At this point the doctors are saying it's NOT a tumor –nor are they saying it's full MS. This may be a one-time event. She's going to start steroid treatments for a few weeks then get another MRI and see where we go from there. While not great, it's the best diagnosis at this point we can hope for, certainly better than some of the other things it could be, so keep your fingers crossed and keep saying prayers. I will touch base with everyone throughout the weekend.

Cooper

Sally wears her emotions on her face; there is never a mystery about what is going on inside her. About 30 minutes into the IV drip she looked at me with those familiar whipped puppy dog eyes.

"What?" I asked.

"I don't want MS," she said.

"It's treatable, and depending on what this is, there are a number of options. But for today, this is the first step and that's what we deal with. Just take it one step at a time." My first attempt at overt caregiving was greeted with a look that if a harpoon gun had been within reach, I'd have been sitting there with a spear implanted in my throat.

So much for successful caregiving. I had much to learn.

What am I feeling right now - besides fear:

_____
_____
_____
_____
_____
_____
_____
_____
_____
_____
_____
_____

The action I will take is:

_____
_____
_____
_____
_____
_____
_____

Notes:

Caregiver Tip #3

Stop looking up everything on the Internet

DIS-information rules on the net. It will cause you more stress and panic than it will calm your fears. You have questions? Ask a doctor, or a nurse, or talk to someone in a support group who has been there before. When it comes to cancer caregiving, with the exception of one or two caregiving sites (*see Appendix A*), the web is just that - a sticky place to get trapped that will come to a bad ending.

One of the benefits of being a control freak is needing to know... everything, and what better place to excavate information than the Internet.[1] Grabbing my smartphone, I tapped my way onto the highway and discovered the steroids Sally was ingesting were not anabolic but dexamethasone, an anti-inflammatory steroid used to decrease swelling associated with tumors of the spine and brain.

Wait a minute. Tumors? No one said anything about tumors. In fact, Dr. Mazlin specifically discounted tumors. Further reading proved just as alarming once I scrolled to the section on side-effects: depression, mood swings, cramps, seizures, vomit that looks like coffee grounds...

Jesus. What else weren't they telling us? I kept my mouth shut, however, not wanting to alarm Sally. I pushed the fear of witnessing any of those events into a deep corner and resolved to just keep watch at all times.

I still had not come to grips with the information-internet issue and searched for ADEM online. Complications such as seizures and coma were listed along with diagnosis activities like getting an MRI...and a lumbar puncture. What the hell was that? Another search revealed this was a fancy name for a spinal tap. That raised a whole new level of fear for me -- and I wasn't even the recipient. In my mind spinal taps were ugly, painful things. My imagination created horrible scenes of pain and torture repeating endlessly in my head.

---

[1] In the dictionary, see Sarcasm.

It didn't occur to me at that time, but I was replaying a familiar scenario, only this time from the inside and not as an observer who could see the consequences. My mom was diagnosed with ovarian cancer, and all during her treatment she kept an encyclopedic book listing all known prescription drugs along their side-effects. Every time her oncologist prescribed a medication, she looked it up in her book, saw the side effects, and decided she would not take the drug.

My sister Joanne, thankfully, finally took the book away from her and said she was going to do what the doctor said and not look up every single drug prescribed.

Eventually it dawned on me that every bit of information I saw online constituted worst-case-scenario thinking that did nothing but increase my panic and anxiety. What solidified my decision to stop referring to online data was a coffee mug.

Upon entering the waiting area of Dr. Tsarouhas' office for my quarterly checkup, I saw a coffee mug at the reception window, used as a pen and pencil holder, with the following words printed on it:

My medical degree outweighs your internet search.

People/Professionals I can call to get questions answered:

_____
_____
_____
_____
_____
_____
_____
_____
_____
_____
_____
_____
_____
_____

Other Important Contacts:

_____
_____
_____
_____
_____
_____
_____

Notes:

Caregiver Tip #4

Adjust your life to allow space for cancer.

Even though you feel like your world has come to a screeching halt, the rest of the planet feels otherwise and will continue on its merry way regardless of your wishes. Some adjustment is called for here. Making space for CANCER in your already jam-packed life will take some, mostly uncomfortable, adjustment. Life's priorities have shifted on you without your consent. Take the time to re-organize: drop what is not critical,

ASK FOR HELP
(where you can)

and realize tasks that were once high on your priority list might have to take a backseat for awhile.

Even though Sally appeared to be on the mend, my inner radar was on full alert twenty-four- seven as I waited for any symptom to reappear signaling a full blown shift into panic mode: if she struggled for a word, or tremors appeared in her hands or arms, bizarre word replacement crept in, or the crash of falling utensils or shattering glassware.

The cause is unclear, but Sally and I have always compressed significant events in our lives into overlapping timelines. Our initial foray into complete insanity occurred during the eighth month of Sally's first pregnancy when we bought our first house and adopted a three-month-old puppy.

So it came as no surprise that Sally's health issues surfaced while we were in the midst of a major real estate transaction – buying a new house, and moving out of a townhouse containing twenty-seven years of memories and enough junk for five dumpsters. With the kids grown and gone and Sally not working, we decided to cut down my sixty-plus minute commute and find a place to live closer to the office.

Traditionally, once empty nesting sets in, most people downsize from their expansive houses to a smaller condo or townhouse. Naturally, we did the opposite. We were planning on going from a townhouse into a three-bedroom, single family home. We continued to enforce everyone's firm belief that we were out of our minds.

Five days before closing on both the new house and the townhouse, we discovered something…

TERMITES.[1]

After requesting a termite inspection, the seller's attorney took the position of "Tough. Deal with it." We took the position of flipping her off and walked away - much to the chagrin of the real estate agents watching their commissions crumble.

In addition to all this came the realization:

"Hey…in three days we're homeless!!"

Simultaneously, and just for laughs, I tried to chop off some fingers by mishandling a bathroom mirror that refused to bend the way I wanted. The laws of physics prevailed, and a large Vermont shaped hunk of jagged glass tried to guillotine my hand.

In answer to crashing glass in the bathtub, I heard Sally scream from downstairs, "Are you okay?". How many answers were there?

"No!" I yelled, looking at my hand's ripped flesh and welling blood.

Wrapping my hand in ice and a wet towel quickly turning red from within, we headed for our frequent hangout of late, Princeton Medical Center at Plainsboro. At least this time we were not going for Sally. Several stitches later, we left the ER and returned to a bathtub of jagged broken glass and the clock continuing to tick, inching closer to not having a roof over our heads.

In our search for temporary lodgings, we discovered that few hotels extend their overnight welcome mat to domesticated quadrupeds, and for those that do, the invitation is only to a select criteria of specific breeds. Any four-legged, flea-circus too large to fit inside a personally monogrammed Coach shoulder bag was deemed unfit to carry the ice bucket through the hotel corridors. With two seventy-pound, rescue bull terrier boxers in tow, our living options were whittled down to a refrigerator packing crate or <u>Extended Stay </u>America.

---

1 In the new house. Our townhouse was pristine, naturally. We hoped.

This particular ESA was not the ideal corporate travel stopover; it was more of a way-station for those with only a vague idea of where their next destination lay. I expected to pass Jack Reacher in the corridor. The facility was set-back off a 60-mile per hour state highway and was surrounded by unlit, wooded grounds. All that was missing was a blinking neon sign reading, Bates Motel. A quick stroll around the premises left me hoping that a limited number of hotel guests fell into the serial killer category.

We moved in on the Thursday before Labor Day weekend, spent ten minutes unpacking a few meager possessions, and then realized we were staring at four full days with absolutely nothing to do.

We spent the unofficial final weekend of summer binge-watching *The First 48* [2], listening for multi-car pileups on Route One, and feeling our anxiety grow; anticipating the follow-up neurology appointment just one week away. Our fervent hope was the steroid treatments did their thing. Imagining the alternatives made my stomach churn and my teeth ache.

On the plus side of hotel living there was no mortgage to pay, no utility bills stuffing the mailbox, and, thankfully, a dearth of home repair chores. On the other hand, Sally, me and the two mouth-breathing, floor-walkers moved into a room half the size of a Manhattan studio apartment, one floor above another long-term guest who let their cat freely roam the halls and stairways. Taking the dogs for a walk made for several re-enactments of classic Tom and Jerry chase scenes.

During the first week of residency, family and friends visited more to gawk at our lodgings than check up on our health. Upon entering our room, the color usually drained from their faces as they went bug-eyed seeing our 200 square foot home, complete with closet-sized kitchenette,

---

2 Our TV choices were limited: the four major networks, one PBS station, QVC, Telemundo, A&E and a local channel dedicated to the intricacies of fishing in the Delaware River in order to catch, gut, and pan-fry some mutant form of grouper.

walls decorated in a lovely institutional green motif, and green and white pseudo-paisley carpeting straight out of a 1955 photo shoot in Better Homes & Gardens.

The night before the follow-up appointment with Dr. Mazlin, we laid in bed and listened to each second tick by, in between the rumbling 18-wheelers that rocketed down Route One, each of us wishing time would speed up; the anticipation of getting some answers was on the one hand a good thing, versus what those answers could be.

After minimal sleep we awoke on September 8, 2014 and celebrated our 35th wedding anniversary by re-visiting the Sesame Place Amusement Park. The Muppets still smiled down from their water-tank perch as we wound back through the smaller, school-is-back-in-session crowds.

We sat in Dr. Mazlin's waiting room reminding ourselves to breathe through the crushing apprehension. Reading outdated issues of People Magazine didn't improve our state and neither was being forced to withstand The View blaring from the omnipresent waiting room flatscreen. I'm unclear what the intended calming effect on a gathering of nervous patients is while held captive and exposed to people screaming at each other. The same was true for nearly every medical office we visited. The latest paranoia from CNN was supposed to make me feel better? At least show something funny; perhaps old Marx Brothers movies or tapes of Richard Nixon resigning.

Once we were summoned to an examination room, Dr. Mazlin brought up the new MRI pictures on his computer, which was wild once I detached myself from the meaning behind them, and realized I was staring at electronic slices of Sally's brain. "In comparing these results to the previous MRI some of the lesions have disappeared," Dr.Mazlin said. A sliver of hope started forming inside me but was quickly dashed.

"However, some new ones have formed. Also, the one that was larger than all the others has increased in size a bit."

The disappointment was palpable on Sally's face. I could see all her hope had been crushed. I'm not sure how successful I was at maintaining any sort of brave face.

He continued. "I've made an appointment for you with Dr. Kastle[3] at Philadelphia General Hospital[4]. He's considered one of the best MS experts in the country. I want to get his opinion on this to confirm my opinion that this is MS."

Happy Anniversary.

So now in addition to living in Motel Hell, we had to travel to Philadelphia to see yet another doctor. In my head this crossed a big line, one that required serious adjustment. Getting treated "locally" held a certain amount of comfort that we remained low on the Serious Medical Condition scale. Somehow moving to Doctors "in the city" significantly boosted the level on that scale and expanded the scary diagnosis possibilities. Thus far, I felt as if we were hamsters stuck on the spinning wheel of unanswered questions. I was running low on strength and resolve, but I took a deep breath, shoved all the fear in some dark place inside and carried on.

After the initial visit with Dr. Kastle in Philly, more blood tests were scheduled two weeks down the road, with a spinal tap scheduled two weeks after that. No one seemed to be in much of a hurry, at least at this point. That was soon to change.

The maddening waiting game dragged on. We reluctantly accepted September's bizarre new routine – spending free time in a hotel king-sized

---

[3] Not a real name. Well, it could be a real name, but it's not THIS doctor's name. You get the idea.
[4] Not a real place that I know of. If it is, just ignore it.

bed, commuting new routes to work, trying to stretch our limited wardrobe to avoid laundry issues.

Sally finally threw in the towel at work. The constant anxiety of not being able to keep up wasn't worth the effort. Even with the MRI results providing photographic proof of the shenanigans messing with her brain, we didn't put two and two together to think "Ahh, this is why work is such a struggle."

Three weeks of hotel life later, closing day on the new house finally arrived. All I was hoping for was a day of smooth transactions.

Bright and early, Sally herded the dogs into her car for a trip to the kennel where they would vacation for a couple days while we unpacked in the new house. Meanwhile I moved our stuff from the hotel room into my car and settled the bill.

Then the phone rang.

It was Sally - in tears. "I had an accident."

"Is everyone okay?" I asked. By this time, she was in tears and was speaking through choking sobs.

"Yes. Nobody…was…hurt." She hit somebody's car at a stop sign. "It wasn't serious, but the guy I hit went nuts screaming at me."

This was Sally's MO; upset first then she'll get pissed later.

Denial showed its ugly face once again: Sally's symptoms had slowly crept back into play, and I had been ignoring them in hopes they just were not real. She had been struggling with words again and now wasn't responding well behind the wheel, both of which ratcheted my fear factor up a couple notches. But I pushed that fear into that same dark inner place that was getting uncomfortably crowded. We were closing today, and I needed to focus on that.

Thankfully, the morning's drama was the only serving of crap for the day. The closing proceeded without a hitch and with hands cramped from signature fatigue we drove, keys in hand, to the new house.

On the one hand, we had a great new house in a town we liked, we were leaving the hotel, and we were getting more stoked about our 40th high school reunion which was a month away. According to the most recent Facebook post, over 130 people had already purchased tickets; a get together at a favorite watering hole was scheduled for Friday night and a Sunday morning breakfast was planned.

On the other hand, we still didn't know what was going on with Sally, our daughter was going through a contentious separation in which Sally was fully entrenched - moms are only has happy as their most miserable kid - and we had a house to unpack amidst all the other new home responsibilities.

Nonetheless, opening the door to the new house, we walked inside for the first time as owners and felt good; an immense post-hotel sigh of relief settled through both of us even with a million boxes to unpack. We were about to get some semblance of our lives back, even if was just access to our "stuff." At this point, any form of familiarity and comfort was welcome.

What can I adjust in my current schedule:
_____
_____
_____
_____
_____
_____
_____
_____
_____
_____
_____
_____

The action I will take is:
_____
_____
_____
_____
_____
_____
_____

Notes:

Caregiver Tip #5

Maintain an Attitude of Gratitude. Things could be worse....

It's easy to become angry and bitter about, well, everything, especially when the patient is suffering. The best way to quell that anger is gratitude. Sometimes the caregiver has to look hard to find the tiniest of things that bring a positive light to the situation, but the search is worth it. Look for ways to be grateful even in the midst of all the stress, fear and anxiety. Even if it's just gratitude at being vertical and breathing for one more day. Keeping an attitude of gratitude, while not always effortless, does make the journey a bit easier.

The following scenes of gratitude break the narrative flow established thus far, but this is such a critical aspect of Caregiver (and patient) mental heath and well-being that grouping them in one place felt appropriate.

Tapped Out Trooper

To say we were not looking forward to the spinal tap is an understatement. Officially this procedure is called a Lumbar Puncture, which for me was not much of an improvement over Spinal Tap, in fact aside from being a great name for a Heavy Metal band, Lumbar Puncture sounded even more painful.

Being new and thoroughly uninformed, the images I was conjuring about the procedure featured extreme horrors of pain as some sadistic surgical wonk went after Sally's spine with a pickaxe.

Dr. Kastle, a short, turtle-headed, academic type, complete with bow tie and a Napoleon complex, provided little solace. While his clinical sales pitch for the spinal tap was reasonable and made diagnostic sense —gathering cellular level information found only in spinal fluid in order to make an accurate diagnosis - his delivery had all the warmth and charm of Ben Stein taking attendance:

"Bueller? Bueller?..."

The spinal tap was scheduled to happen the week before our class reunion, and we were assured there would be no complications that would prevent us from attending.

In truth, there should not have been.

Dr. Kastle's waiting area at Philly General had "Welcome to the Department of Motor Vehicles" stamped all over it; a minimum of five receptionists sat lined up along the length of a never ending room while less than happy people were scattered around, sitting on institutional chairs and waiting for their numbers to be called - not exactly that warm, Saturday Evening Post feeling of the Norman Rockwell doctor's office.

Once checked in, Sally and I sat in terrified silence. As the patient, Sally was the guinea pig here; she was the one imagining what sort of pain this medieval-sounding medical practice was going to bring her.[1] For me, I was in full protection mode with little I could do to fulfill that role. Additionally, I was the one who had to keep an eye on her once we were home, and I had no idea what to look for should anything go wrong.

So, we sat, holding hands and staring into space, feeling like every second lasted three hours.

A century later a young, white coated, Asian gentleman with tousled black hair, steel-rimmed specs and a smiling face sauntered into the waiting area calling, "Sally Cooper?"

She took a deep breath and stood, giving me one last glance, hoping I had something to impart to her to provide solace. I just smiled. It was the best I could muster.

I aged a dozen years sitting in the waiting area. Being a control freak, turning over people I care about into the hands of strangers to endure actions I knew nothing about made me as uneasy as a cockroach scurrying down Broadway on a Saturday night.. I felt a pang of guilt as I took some comfort in remaining in the waiting room instead of the one being tapped.

Not 30 minutes later, Sally and her escort sauntered back in the room, chatting amiably, as if they had just finished a pleasant lunch and a stroll in the park. Sally looked…fine. Not beaten up or ghostly white. I was able to breathe again.

As a burgeoning caretaker, I had done my spinal tap research. The unanimous consensus was that the patient should be on their back for a brief period of time immediately following the procedure to allow the puncture to heal.

"Okay, so what now?" I asked the technician. "Does she have to be on her back the rest of the day?"

---

[1] What's next? Leeches?

He replied, his smile never wavering, "No. There's really no evidence that staying on your back is necessary. Just take it easy for the rest of the day, no lifting, no driving, nothing strenuous and you should be fine." This flew in the face of everything I had read so my skepticism grew. But, I reasoned, their spinal tap experience outweighed mine so I rolled with it.

The next day, Saturday, Sally's primary goal for the day was finding a dress for the reunion, which was exactly one week away. I have yet to come across any ancient text or constitutional amendment stating new dresses at special events are a requirement, but through some unwritten law none of the 50 dresses in the closet would suffice. It is also an unwritten law that these special event dresses, regardless of how well they fit or make her look, will be returned after the event has passed. I've spent hours and hours trying to figure out what the dresses in the closet represent in light of the special event dress cycle, I've thought about it and thought about it until I popped a brain aneurism. I concluded that this was a law of female nature and that acceptance was better than understanding.

Sally took off early Saturday morning and I cocooned myself back in bed. Twenty minutes later, half conscious, I was startled awake by the slam of the back door. I thought, there's no way she found a dress that quickly. Buying a new dress was at least a two to three store excursion. She entered the bedroom and the first thing I noticed was that her face had taken on a reptilian shade of green. Without a word she crawled into bed, turned on her back and stared at the ceiling. I knew that look, intense focus to keep from puking.

"What's going on?" I asked.

She held up a hand – the international signal for

If-I-Answer-You-Now-I'm-Going-To-Hurl - Ask-Me-Later.

Once the shade of green morphed into something paler I got the story.

"I had to pull off the road to get sick," she said quietly. "I got dizzy and nauseous all of a sudden. The vertigo didn't go away so I came home." My stomach lurched. Sally's driving skills were already impaired. With vertigo added... I said a quick prayer of thanks to whatever force got her home safely.

My first reaction? Call in the professionals. Then it hit me; Saturday - the professionals would be few and far between, a thought which proved accurate after calling Dr. Kastle's office attempting to track down anyone on the MS staff at the hospital. No one was there. Nor was our neurologist, Dr. Mazlin, available. Why does this shit always happen on a weekend?

Striking out phone-wise, I checked on Sally who was still on her back, but fast asleep. I thought about heading to the hospital ER, but there was something that kept me from taking that route. This was a spinal tap, not a sliced finger. Plus I really did not want to move Sally without someone telling me what the hell was going on.

Sally woke a couple hours later. Some color had returned, and she said she felt better, not light-headed, just drained. Good signs, we agreed, so prone in bed was the course of action for the remainder of Saturday and Sunday. Come Monday we would call Dr. Kastle's office and get their take on the whole thing. I still had no idea what was going on, but as long as Sally was feeling better, I could breathe a little easier. Denial kept me thinking that since whatever happened was not getting any worse, then no immediate action was required.[2]

By Sunday night Sally was able to sit up in bed without the room spinning and actually eat something without it making a return appearance. My tension and fear eased a bit further.

---

2 No medical school for me, thanks.

On Monday I called Dr. Kastle's office at Philadelphia General, told the receptionist what was going on, and that we needed some direction. She took my info and said someone would get back to me.

In the meantime, Sally was feeling progressively better; she was moving around the house in short bursts without any ill effects and was eating normally.

In the face of the unknown without any reliable assistance, I can make my own diagnoses. While I was happy that Monday ended uneventfully, I was more than slightly pissed that I did not get a return call from Dr. Kastle's office.

By Tuesday morning Sally was about 75% normal, feeling good, doing some light stuff around the house. Finally, Tuesday afternoon we got a return call from one of Dr. Kastle's minions, saying that it sounded like whatever had happened had corrected itself and to just keep activity to a minimum for a while. If anything else happened, we were to let them know. Comforting.

Sally's positive progress continued through the week. By Friday, she was back to form, taking the dog for a short walk, and talking about the reunion. The original dress dilemma remained unsolved, and the reunion was 24 hours away. We agreed, given the week's activities, that we would skip the Friday night classmate get together in Westfield; that it might be too much of a push and we did not want to jeopardize getting to the reunion the next day. To play it safe, Sally stayed home on Friday but would go out Saturday morning in search of something to wear. We were confident that we had trudged our way through the unexpected crisis, and our anticipation was high for the following night's long-awaited get together.

Finally, Reunion Saturday. As she did the week before, Sally got up early and headed out in search of a dress.

As I did the week before, I rolled over in bed, only this time sleep was elusive as anticipation was high and faces from 40 years past churned through my brain. I felt as if I was going home after an extended absence, reuniting with people who meant so much, wondering how their lives had changed over the past four decades. Letting all the memories of school comfort me like wearing the most comfortable t-shirt and jeans I owned. I smiled to myself, thinking about…

Then, just like the week before, the back door slammed.

Twenty seconds later, Sally was back in bed, garbage can at her side.

"Same thing? I asked tentatively.

"Same," she said, not wanting to speak further for fear of puking yet again.

I let her sleep and realized it was Saturday once again - reaching out to Dr. Kastle's office was futile.

In exasperation, I called our family doctor, who had given us his direct cell phone number for emergencies.

After I explained what had happened over the past week or so, he said, "She needs a blood patch. No question. I'm just not qualified to perform it. You'll have to wait until Monday when the Philadelphia doctor is available."

I wanted to rip out somebody's eyeballs and grind them in the kitchen disposal. No way in hell was Sally going to make the reunion. I was not going to leave her on her own and go by myself. Crushed. What was bliss had turned to complete heartbreak in a matter of seconds.

Researching "blood patch" online,[3] I found out that it was a procedure in which blood is extracted from the patient and then placed over the leaking hole in the outer layer covering the spine, the hole that was made to extract the spinal fluid.

If that initial puncture never heals, the fluid leaks and never reaches the brain, thus the feelings of vertigo and nausea.

There was little solace in that knowledge except that I now knew what was going on in Sally's body.

She slept most of the day. I sat around getting more angry and depressed. At around five in the afternoon, we talked about what would happen next.

"We are staying here," I said, feeling as discouraged as the look on Sally's face.

From her prone bed position she said, "You go."

"No. I'm not going without you, and you need to stay here until we get this taken care of."

An hour later I went back upstairs to see if Sally needed anything. The sight of an empty bed was more than alarming. Panicked, I dashed to the bathroom, but instead of catastrophe I found her standing at the bathroom mirror applying mascara.

"What are you doing?" I said in disbelief.

"I feel better. We're going."

I knew she was trying hard to rally, I wasn't sure it was a good idea. "I'm not buying it," I said.

"Cooper, we have to go. I'll be fine." Torpedo in the water.

"I'm still not buying it," which I felt was what I was supposed to say. Inside I felt a spark of hope ignite but was trying to keep that under wraps.

---

[3] Special dispensation of internet usage - just looking up technical info not symptoms or side effects.

"Let's go," she said, "and if I start to feel shitty, we'll leave. We have to go. Even if it's just for an hour or two."

Sally was pushing, trooper that she was. If I had felt as bad as she did, I would not have mustered the courage to move from the bed and soldier on.

I was torn. My logical side knew the sensible thing to do was to bag the reunion and stay home. My inner child was starting to perform cartwheels.

As we got dressed, I kept a wary eye on Sally, looking for any signs of faltering. I knew that she was not magically better, given the past week's events. Deep inside I knew this was a temporary reprieve, a small window Sally opened that could slam shut at any moment.

The trip to the venue wasn't exactly a five-minute ride, more like an hour plus, and I was conscious of every bump we hit along the way.

Once we arrived, I'm sure Sally was sick to death of me asking "Are you okay?"

Sally appeared to be holding her own, upbeat, smiling – truly enjoying herself -- even though in my gut I knew we were on borrowed time. I was in awe of the courage she showed going from being a walking ad for vertigo to full-press partying.

At the two-hour mark, we sat at one of the large round tables talking with old friends. I glanced to my right, and I saw Sally's eyes glaze over in a vacant stare. She was done.

"Come on. Let's go," I said softly. She nodded in agreement. After waiting 15 minutes for her to emerge from the bathroom, we quickly bundled up and headed home, Sally with a plastic bag in the front seat retching her guts out for most of the ride.

"Trooper" is too lame a word for her. The fact that she extracted her head from the bedside puke bucket and bulled her way through the feelings of dizziness and nausea to allow us the treat of even a small amount of time at the reunion was above and beyond the call. I wanted to wave a magic wand and make it all go away for her. Harry Potter I'm not, but my gratitude was boundless.

She spent Sunday in bed. On Monday I called Dr. Kastle's office, and with a few ugly words about availability and responsible information, the nurse said, matter-of-factly, "Just go to your local ER and get a blood patch."

Seriously. Are you fucking kidding me?

We went, once again, to Princeton Medical Center.[4] Blood patch done, 1, 2, 3. Back home, a day of rest and she was fine. Sally went through nine days of hell for this, and the Philadelphia General staff acted as if she did nothing more than skin her knee.

I vowed to strike them off my Christmas card list.

Pinheads.

Take A Look Around

"Come on," I said jumping off the bed, "Grab your I.V. stand, and let's go for a walk."

Even a minor change of scenery can help lift some of the rotten feelings of a cancer patient, not to mention the caregiver as well, and while this was not exactly a stroll up 5th Avenue to gaze at the holiday decorated windows, it would suffice. We made three round trips around the corridor, which took approximately five minutes. On the fourth lap, I leaned closer to Sally and whispered, "You know, judging by some of the other patients on this floor, we could be a lot worse off than we are. Some of these people are really struggling."

"I know. I've noticed that."

---

[4] The Jim and Sally Cooper Trauma Center at Princeton Medical Center is scheduled to open in 2027

As we walked around the hospital corridor, we realized how much worse our situation could be. There were so many people getting treatment that are two-, three- and four-time repeaters: breast cancer, colon cancer, stomach cancer, throat cancer, and yet, they keep their own hopes alive through all the surgeries, all the treatments and all the time alone.

A spoonful of gratitude helps you snap out of the doldrums pretty damn quick.

Take A Closer Look Around

I had to sleep under Sally's bed during the fifth round of chemo.

Well, sort of.

We were stationed in a corner room and while the views were outstanding and the room, as a whole, was larger than the hallway rooms, the space was divided horizontally instead of vertically, which meant the floor space for my transformed sleeper chair was reduced to less than the width of the chair itself; I slept with the dividing shower curtain hanging over me. It also meant all staff and visitors had to climb through patient A's quadrant to reach patient B. We were patient A.

Patient B and her partner made their grand entrance around two in the morning, just as I was finally starting to doze. Patient B was not a happy camper and sounded like she was continually drowning in her own sputum. Patient B's partner only added to the carnage, flailing the divider curtains, using the patient bathroom, talking at full volume.

After an hour of grinding my teeth and trying to maintain patience, I reached my breaking point.

Out in the hallway I tracked down Sally's nurse, Michee – the first and only time the poor young lady was assigned to us.

"This is not going to work," I said as calmly as possible. Michee knew what I was talking about, I could see it in her eyes. Nurses and nurse managers attempted to explain the facts of life to patient B's partner and made an attempt to relieve the patient of whatever was going on.

By half-past three things settled down, with the prospect of the first herd of doctors making their first rounds in a couple hours.

By the third day exhaustion was wreaking havoc with Sally and me, our patience honed razor thin, and in the grips of February cabin fever. The honeymoon phase of treatment had worn off completely.

With lunch finished in the cafeteria, I headed back to the ugly prospect of an afternoon enduring thoroughly annoying and ineffective conference calls at work. I felt myself itching for a fight, not the optimal frame of mind to bring to the corporate table. Scowling, I climbed on the elevator.

"Hold, please!" a woman's voice off to the side, out of my field of vision. I thought, "Jesus. Come on already."

A young mom appeared, haggard and drawn, pushing a wheelchair containing a little girl, not more than seven or eight, hairless, wearing a surgical mask and attached to several IV bags hung from the stand welded to the chair. Mom maneuvered her daughter into the cramped car.

"Where to?" I asked. The girl gave me the floor that represented the children's cancer section.

At that moment, all the mundane irritants I thought were so critical popped into nothingness like a balloon hitting a porcupine. I pushed the button and looked, surreptitiously I hoped, at the little girl in the wheelchair. What she was enduring is something no child should have to. In my mind I wondered how this had come to pass, that children who don't yet know what life is about find themselves battling to keep breathing one more day. One day at a time. And yet maintain a smile and a sparkle in their eye.

"How's it going?" I asked. I figured I better say something instead of just rudely staring.

"Okay, I guess. I have a couple more treatments before I'll know for sure," she said, the outline of a smile underneath her mask.

"You hang tough," I said. I looked at Mom, who had a weak smile and the perpetual glassy-eyed stare of a helpless parent watching their child suffer.

My perspective made a one-eighty. The afternoon was calm now that the storm of self-involvement had passed.

I realized the people who traveled the cancer highway had two choices: face it with hope and gratitude or face it with bitter resentment and anger. Everyone chooses their own approach and there are plenty within each group.

Experiencing the living proof of faith and courage in the positive survivors who engage in battle after battle, and seeing the unthinkable solutions and treatments available, my daily work tasks became no more significant than a puddle after a rainstorm, dealing with the drama of ensuring software operated efficiently to allow a salesperson to sell a ten dollar cell phone case.

Looking into that young girl's eyes, at the very heart of courage, reminded me of another courageous mother and child much closer to my heart.

Touchstones

In the summer of 2000, I met Donya, this punk kid with the attitude of a 40-year-old and a Yahtzee celebration dance that, if I had tried to imitate it, would have ruptured three discs and caused internal bleeding. I was 44, she was 20, but we connected through an intense healing journey that we travelled together. Fourteen years later, during my Facebook initiation,

I found her again, only this time she was married and had a three-year-old daughter who was about to undergo an historic liver transplant in order to combat a disease so rare there were only eight cases of it in existence in the world. I was able to see how Donya coped or didn't, as happened on occasion. Here was someone coming face-to -ace with life threatening clouds hanging over her baby. Donya became a touchstone; I thought of her every time I started feeling sorry for myself; thought of the bottomless well of strength she relied on while her young daughter battled to stay alive.

The courage and strength of others worked wonders in bolstering my gratitude for all the blessings bestowed upon us thus far.

Things for which I am grateful:

_____
_____
_____
_____
_____
_____
_____
_____
_____
_____
_____
_____

Actions of gratitude I can take:

_____
_____
_____
_____
_____
_____
_____
_____

Notes:

Caregiver Tip #6

Trust your instincts.
Tune into the *gentle* voice in your head; it will guide you where you need to go.

In the absence of fact, or when you are torn making critical decisions, trust the voice in your head. The gentle one, not the one that talks you down and screams at you. The one that feels reassuring.

We nervously made our way to Philadelphia General to finally, after four weeks, get the results of all the bloodwork and the spinal tap. Both of us were sizzling with anxiety like an overhead electric wire ripped loose and snaking wildly in the air. We entered Dr. Kastle's examination room and was surprised to see him deeply engaged in conversation with a dark-haired young woman in a white lab coat, someone we had never met before.

As if realizing Sally and I had somehow just materialized in the room, Kastle said, "Do you mind if my medical intern is present? This is part of her required training."

I found this odd, considering the possibilities of what the test results might tell us, but we raised no objections. I supposed interns had to get their hands-on training somewhere.

Dr. Kastle continued to address the intern, talking about process and procedure. After a minute, and without so much as taking a breath, and with all the warmth, subtlety, and finesse of a Megadeath concert, the doctor turned to us and said, "It's lymphoma," and without the slightest change in demeanor, returned his attention to his young protégée.

I'm not sure whose jaw hit the floor first, but I became instantly stone deaf; not a single sound could break through the shock and screaming in my brain. Sally's expression revealed that someone had just ripped out her heart and soul – vacant but incredulous.

In that moment, our lives changed irrevocably; with the utterance of a single word, everything we had assumed would happen, living comfortably to old age with the usual aches and pains, retiring somewhere nice, watching our kids and grandkids grow and prosper, enjoying friends and life with a sense of peace and fulfillment, was instantly wiped out; we had new lives to lead. Every decision going forward would have

Cancer

mixed into the process.

Ever see the horror movie *Species*? There's a scene where the evil creature reaches into a woman's body and yanks out her spine. Doctor Turtlehead dove at us with both hands and came away with a spine in each hand.

I finally said, "Excuse me?"

He replied as if reading off a restaurant menu. "It's B cell lymphoma. You'll need to have a brain biopsy and begin chemotherapy. I've already contacted the neurosurgeon upstairs as all this needs to be done fairly quickly."

Oh, so now speed was of the essence. Asshat.

He continued. "I'm going to take you to meet him now."

We piled in the elevator with Dr. Kastle, I fought to maintain control and not run screaming from the building; it was up to me to stay focused on what these clowns were telling us as I knew Sally was thoroughly out of commission, in a total state of disbelief with no communication skills. Numbness prevented either of us from making a move to comfort the other; holding hands, a hug, let alone speak. We stood in the elevator's back corners, using the walls to keep us from collapsing into a heap on the floor. What I really wanted to do was take a flat wooden paddle scrawled with the Hippocratic Oath and beat Dr. Kastle senseless. I resisted.

We were dumped unceremoniously into yet another waiting room and Kastle departed. That was the last we ever saw of him.

We sat in the waiting area, looking newly lobotomized, staring into space. Eventually the neurosurgeon strolled in. He had a physique conducive to juggling 18-wheeler diesel transmissions for fun and bench-pressing Chryslers just for the hell of it; big son of a gun. He started regurgitating how the process would go and that we would need to get the biopsy done quickly so chemo could start. His presentation evinced an attitude indicating that he would shoot himself if he had to give this speech one more time. I wondered if lack of personality was a requirement for medical practice at Philly General. Maybe if I took all of them out for a cheesesteak and a beer, things might loosen up a bit.

I didn't hear every word but through my stupefaction I was cognizant enough to get the gist of what he was saying – biopsy and chemo. Got it. Sally was stone silent. Shock tends to have that effect.

Everything was moving too fast. A mountain of information assaulted us, assessing it all felt insurmountable, as did breathing normally.

"Wait," I said, "We need to talk about this overnight. Just to digest it all. We can call you in the morning to let you know how we want to proceed." I knew we didn't have much choice, but I was not going to commit to anything without a chance to regain my equilibrium. I assumed Sally felt the same, if not worse.

"That's fine," he said. "But don't put this off. This is an aggressive form of cancer and needs attention."

No shit.

The drive home was punctuated with a deafening silence, and a large amount of disbelief. We got home, still said little, and ate less. We went to bed knowing any attempt at sleep would provide fitful results at best. The one thing we agreed on was keeping the news to ourselves for the time being. Family and friends would be apprised once we had a chance to put all the pieces together.

Laying in bed, I grew increasingly agitated with how all this went down at the hospital. Aside from getting the news from Tooter the Turtle,[1] the whole Philly vibe didn't feel right. In the deep distance of my brain, a voice was trying to break through the slog, a voice that was speaking the truth of what I was feeling. Over the years I have learned to trust this voice but, at that moment, I didn't hear what it was saying.

Cancer. What the hell was I supposed to do with that? How was I going to make sure Sally got the care she needed when I didn't know the first thing about it and had zero support network for this stuff? I like to lean on trusted experts when I can, if for no other reason than to bolster my confidence that whatever action I take is the right thing. In this case I felt lost, as if the weight of this decision rested squarely with me. Oncology doctors were not in my network of acquaintances, and I did not know anyone who had experienced this type of cancer. I needed solid information, especially when it came to explaining to our kids and the rest of the family what was happening. I knew they would have the same questions I did and a few more I didn't.

Fear. About making the wrong decision, about screwing up in the eyes of others, about Sally not getting better. How the hell was I going to keep control on the situation without losing my mind?

The next morning, Sally and I lay in bed wondering if either of us had bothered to record the license plate of the 18-wheeler that had plowed into us. This really wasn't happening, was it? Up until now cancer was something that happened to other people but certainly not to us. I was scared and confused. Additionally, the sterile nature of the good folks

---

1 If you were not a child of the sixties glued to Saturday morning cartoons, just Google this name. That's easier than trying to explain it.

at Philly General left me feeling suspicious and pissed off. We were in a life-threatening area with zero experience.

The information and the source of that information was something I had to trust and thus far, Dr. Kastle and Company had done little to win that trust. But what other choice was there?

"I guess I better call them," I said, "are you okay with that?"

Still somewhat in shock, Sally nodded, a look of absolute terror in her eyes.

Mobile phone in hand, I tapped out the neurosurgeon's number, but hesitated before hitting the green send button. I just stared at the phone.

My inner voice was begging for attention; like a kid chasing a departing ice cream truck, screaming at it to stop. It was keeping my hand in paralysis, keeping me from tapping the green call button. I continue to stare at the phone. Deep inside a spark grew - call it confidence, call it a force - but the growing sensation that a different path was needed started taking root…and it felt good.

"No," I said out loud, clicking the button to turn off the phone. "This just doesn't feel right. I don't have an answer, but this just can't be the way this is supposed to happen. I'm going to start making phone calls to anyone I can think of to get some help. But going back to Philly feels wrong."

Sally emphatically agreed. Memories of the spinal tap disaster and the diagnosis presentation created the same ill-will I felt.

Okay. So now what? Just making the decision about Philly General felt energizing; the momentum shifted, slightly, to our favor.

Call number one was to my sister-in-law Trish, a career operating room nurse who, I figured, had to have solid contacts in the medical community. It was possible she could steer us in a better direction, and indeed she came through. She had worked with a surgeon in north Jersey with a great reputation and urged us to contact him. I called his office, explained the situation, and left a message for him to return my call.

The next call was to our family doctor Lou Tsarouhas. Again, after explaining the situation, he recommended a neurosurgeon colleague Dr. Nirav Shah.

"If I had to have a brain biopsy, this is the guy I would want doing it," Lou said.

Another call was made to Dr. Shah's office; I recounted the same story and left the same message. As both doctors were recommended by trusted sources, speed would be the decider here; how soon they could see Sally, look at the MRI's and associated data, and give us an opinion.

In the end, visiting Trish's colleague was a two-day wait. Dr. Shah would see us that afternoon. Dr. Shah it was.

Even before the appointment, this decision just felt right. We remained oblivious to what lay ahead, but a vail of fear had eased a bit from both of us, if for no other reason than feeling confident that whatever power had spoken to us and directed us away from Philadelphia was now guiding us in the right direction.

Dr. Shah's waiting area was the opposite of the chrome and fluorescent décor of all the offices we had visited thus far -- warm greens and subdued yellow lighting. Welcoming instead of chilling.

In the absence of Sally's ability to think and write coherently, my next caregiver skill became filling out medical forms. Some of them contained more pages than a Stephen King novel. Once all the formalities were complete, we were led to an examination room. There's not much that can be done with the ambiance of an examination room. It is what it is; I was slowly learning to accept the vinyl covered exam tables with a jumbo roll of waxpaper at the head, and the extra chairs or benches that were a chiropractor's nightmare.

Dr. Shah skateboarded into the examination room with one knee on a chair and the other leg pushing him along. A round-faced, soft-spoken man with gentle eyes that connected to whomever he addressed.

"While this looks like CNS lymphoma, we need to perform a biopsy to confirm," he said, with only a trace of an Indian accent. "My partner, Dr. Josepher, and I will extract some of the cells that are affected and have them analyzed. It still could be several other things, so I don't want to make a final diagnosis until we have the results."

We liked him immediately. He scheduled the biopsy, to be performed at our home away from home, Princeton Medical Center, on November 10th. Dr. Shah's expectation was that Sally would spend a single night in recovery in the hospital and would be discharged the next day. Given this information, Sally had one question...

"Will I get to keep my hair?"

This taught me that women can accept someone taking a cordless Makita drill to their skull, but their biggest concern remains hair loss. The magnitude of this trauma is on par with guys losing their cellphone or watching the Giants blow a fourteen-point lead late in the fourth quarter. I thought it a trivial issue as I live with constant hair loss, but minimizing hair loss would be like telling Sally one of her children wasn't really hers.

Dr. Shah assured her they would shave a small patch, but the rest of her coiffure would be fine.

"One question," I said to Dr. Shah. "Driving."

He didn't even hesitate and directed his answer to Sally. "For now, I don't want you getting behind the wheel. Not until we know exactly what we're dealing with and how it's going to be treated." Sally appeared crestfallen. I breathed an immense sigh of relief. I was not without sympathy. I know someday when I'm old and feeble my license will be revoked and when that happens, send for Dr. Kevorkian.

Regardless, I was able to acknowledge that my gut had steered us in the right direction, that whatever voice reached out to me that prevented me from calling Philly General knew what the hell it was doing. There was one step remaining for final confirmation, and I was confident we had fallen into more than capable hands, which allowed me to wake up each day prior to the surgery without a knot of fear, at least for this phase. What was to come presented its own set of challenges.

Gentle thoughts (the good ones):

_____
_____
_____
_____
_____
_____
_____
_____
_____
_____
_____

Louder thoughts (the not-so-good ones):

_____
_____
_____
_____
_____
_____
_____

Notes:

Caregiver Tip #7

Spirituality. Get some.

It makes little difference if what brings you peace is traditional Judeo-Christian dogma, Buddhism, Druidism, or if you worship aquamarine penguins dancing the merengue. Leaning on the thing that gives you a sense of calm is essential. Use it well, and often.

One would think that listening to my inner voice came as second nature, given recent events. History had certainly provided conclusive evidence. In 2012, after working for 11 years as a contractor for a major telecommunications firm, a nagging notion insisted I become a full time employee. Why then, as opposed to anytime previously, was a mystery – at that time. After months of searching and networking, the company agreed and I graduated into the employee ranks.

Following news of Sally's diagnosis and condition, my employer graciously agreed to allow me to work from home; an act of empathy for which I will be forever grateful, and an inconceivable arrangement were I a contractor. At home, I ensured nothing got out of hand, new symptoms didn't appear, medication dosages were correctly administered, dogs cared for, and friends and family were kept in the loop.

Not to mention working an eight-hour day; endless conference calls, sifting through streaming emails, putting out fires. Then there was my actual work.

In short order, I felt myself starting to run out of steam, physically and emotionally. Come 11 at night, I collapsed in a chair with my insides still driving at 150 miles an hour but without an ounce of energy left, knowing it would easily be one in the morning before sleep entered the picture, while staring at a seven o'clock wake up call to get up and do it all again.

We were still lucky, though. Sally's ability to perform basic self-maintenance wasn't hindered but her decision-making process, the ability to act out of common sense without possible injury to herself or others, resembled Lucy Ricardo on the candy factory assembly line. Her job already showed us that she had trouble handling multiple tasks without being overwhelmed. Simple tasks such as brushing her teeth or bathing posed little threat. My concern was anything involving motor skills and open flame (the stove), heating (the microwave), communications of an emergency nature, or any combination of the above.

10 November 2014. Biopsy day. Trees remained decorated with blinding reds, oranges and yellows with stubborn vestiges of green, and the warm air felt like a holdover from September. Heading to Princeton Medical Center had become as routine as a trip to the grocery store.

Sally's brain surgeon, Dr. Shah entered her room with his colleague Dr. Seth Josepher, a rail-thin, soft-spoken man who appeared as if he would be knocked over by an oscillating fan set on low. Both were dressed in surgeons' green scrubs. Josepher empathetically directed his statements in a soft-spoken tone to Sally without condescension.

"The procedure should take about 20 minutes, and you'll be out of recovery about an hour after that," he said, flashing a confident smile.

When the orderly appeared about 15 minutes later, I looked down into Sally's eyes and conjured up the most reassuring smile I could. What I really wanted to do was grab the gurney and make a mad dash for the exit. Sally's sister Katie stood next to me and watched Sally roll down the hallway into the elevator. We stood, helpless, as the elevator doors closed.

"Ever wanted to jump out of your skin?" I murmured to Katie, still staring at the closed elevator doors as if expecting an encore.

"Oh yeah," she said.

Sitting in an empty hospital room was not going to keep us calm so we headed for the cafeteria and waited. What else was there to do?

Through everything we had experienced thus far, this was the first time I felt completely and totally lost. Two guys whom I had just met were about to dig into my wife's skull. This was not a blood draw or an MRI; the gravity of what was happening behind closed doors hit hard. My role was to sit and wait, like a claustrophobic in a coffin.

"I can't take much more of this," I said. Katie didn't respond.

We sat in the cafeteria watching the clock tick and being scared to death. Eating was out of the question.

Suddenly, from behind me, a voice said, "Mr. Cooper?"

A nurse in green hospital scrubs with a wide Jamaican smile was staring at me so I assumed she was the one who addressed me. It took a minute, but I realized she was the first nurse we met in August to get IV steroid treatments. We had seen her just once, three months earlier, and she not only remembered us, but remembered what Sally was battling. I was floored, and comforted.

She asked, "How is your wife doing?" I explained what was going on with the brain biopsy and that she was with Dr. Shah in surgery.

"He's the best. She's in excellent hands. I will say a prayer for you."

That sort of concern and care was a universe away from what we experienced in Philadelphia. Again, the decision we made to go elsewhere was reinforced. This was the first inkling that whatever force lurked in thecosmos was hard at work and provided what I needed at the moment I needed it.

We walked into Sally's room, post-recovery, and there she was; fragile, unconscious with a big old white gauze bandage slapped on the left side of her head. My heart shattered harder than I ever thought possible. There was a certain part of me that felt responsible; wasn't it my job to protect and keep my loved ones from being hurt and bandaged?

Even though she exacted a promise from Dr. Shah concerning her hair, Sally was not going to be happy that one side of her head had a crop circle shaved into it.

I sat on the edge of the bed. Her eyelids fluttered open as she tried to focus through the anesthesia glaze in her eyes.

"Hi," I said.

She opened her mouth to respond, but nothing came out. She just smiled and closed her eyes.

"Why can't she speak?" I thought in a panic. Had something gone horribly wrong? Losing speech was not part of the Here's-What-To-Expect-Post-Surgery brochure. My first inclination was to press hard on the nurses' call button until the entire staff rushed in with a crash cart to fix whatever the hell was going on. My second inclination was just to jump out of the window. Neither happened. Instead, I just held her hand, smiled, and let her drift back to sleep, all while feeling helpless and stupid that there was nothing else I could do.

Doctors Shah and Josepher entered the room later and assured us that everything went according to plan, there were no complications and that she was fine. They were waiting for the official analysis of the sample they extracted, but they were confident that it was lymphoma. I always imagined that when a doctor approached with the news starting with "we are confident..." that the information that followed would be positive:

> "Mr. Jones, we are confident that Timmy's leg was set completely, and he'll be running again in no time."
>
> "Mrs. Simpson, Bart is in recovery. We are confident we removed all the lug nuts from his colon."

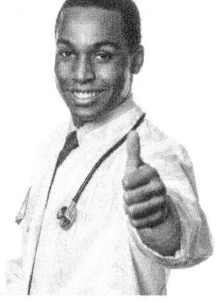

Was I supposed to be overjoyed that they confirmed my wife's head was full of cancer? I made a mental note to start carrying my bottle of Ativan with me at all times, either that or request a bourbon IV drip.

With his impish grin Dr. Josepher gave Sally the once over.

"Sally," he said, after gently jostling her awake, "what is your name?"

She stared at him wide-eyed, but could not produce an answer. I could tell she was giving it serious consideration, and very possibly knew the answer in her head but could not articulate it.

"That's okay," Josepher said, "you're doing fine." To the crowd in the room he said, " She'll stay here tonight, and we should see improvement tomorrow. There's no reason she should not be able to go home then."

Around lunchtime, Josepher pulled me out of the room, and we met Dr. Shah in the family waiting area. The sample analysis confirmed that it was indeed lymphoma.

"Why couldn't she come up with her name?" I asked, "Is that the anesthesia?"

"No," Josepher said. "The air channel created by the burr hole in her skull is causing the speech difficulties. It will dissipate over the next 24 hours as the channel heals over."

I was happy that they agreed to put Sally back on steroids for a limited time until the chemo treatments began.

Then, Dr Shah asked, "Do you know an oncologist you can contact?"

Why not just shoot me with a taser? My brain raced. I thought, why can't you guys do it? I'm feeling comfortable with your care, and now I've got to go to someone else? I was feeling passed around like a church collection plate. How would I know an oncologist unless I'd been down this road before?

Then, whatever guiding force had brought me to this point pushed a bit further, reminding me that I actually had been down this road before.

"Does Dr. Ye still practice?" I asked.

Both Shah and Josepher nodded. "Absolutely. He's one of the best. We will pass all the data over to him and have him call you to set up an appointment."

Dr. Michael Ye had been the archangel oncologist in Princeton who rescued my mom from Hannibal Lecter, the butcher who performed her cancer surgery. Post-surgery, Dr. Lecter announced to the entire waiting room that my mom had had six months to live. Under Dr. Ye's care, my mom plowed her way through another five years of life including a period of total remission. The doctor called her "The Miracle Lady." My panic of once again breaching into the unknown subsided a bit.

By noon the next day, when Dr. Josepher once again asked Sally her name, she was able to produce her maiden name "Sally Howard" as an answer.

Close enough for jazz.

Still wobbly, Sally was dressed in pedestrian clothes and firmly planted in a wheelchair. With hugs from the nurses[1], we wheeled out of the hospital but not before running into an old friend and neighbor, Kate, and her famed therapy Maltipoo Lily, both of whom paid many visits to the hospital bringing some cheer to patients and staff alike. A little spark reignited in Sally's eyes having Lily on her lap and getting a smile and hug from Kate. More evidence; something provided Sally with the right thing at the right time.

Within a week, Sally's stitches were out, and she was sharp again thanks to the anesthesia completely dissipating and the steroid reintroduction.

---

[1] Two days spent mostly unconscious and Sally had bonded with the nurses. Talk about foreshadowing…

To her delight, hair quickly started sprouting on the shaved patch on her head, enough so she could venture outside hatless. I explained the next step to her once she was semi-rational; she was comfortable with seeing Dr. Ye, knowing the care he provided my mom.

Several weeks before she died in 2001, I spent an entire day with Mom, wheelchair-ing her between three different doctor's appointments to get injections, check-ups and more injections.

The last stop for the day was Dr. Ye's office. He was a short man with a round face of pure compassion and a soft-spoken yet direct manner. He spoke the truth to Mom, but with warmth and empathy. Even though it was becoming obvious that Mom was failing by this point, he still referred to her as "The Miracle Lady." He was the first person I witnessed who treat my mom with that sort of compassion; the type of care that leaves an indelible mark.

When Sally and I met with Dr. Ye, his manner had not changed, an encroaching grayness at the temples was attempting to take over his jet-black hair, but that did not detract from his gentle face.

He verified Sally's large B-cell lymphoma and showed us diagrams and factoids from a notebook he had about the cancer, what it does, and how it's treated.

"Using chemotherapy or possibly radiation; this type of lymphoma can be eradicated," he told us.

Then he unloaded the bombshell.

"Unfortunately, I cannot treat it. It is not my area of expertise."

The floor dropped out from under me as I had a sense of what was coming - we were going to be passed off to yet another unknown entity. The calm and good fortune I was feeling was quickly replaced by the all too familiar tension and fear of the unknown.

He continued, "I'm referring you to Dr. Grav, Grove…I can never say it so I call him Dr. G. He is a neurologist at Memorial Sloan Kettering." He produced a business card.

"I see why you stick with Dr. G," I said, doing my best to read the card. Dr. Igor Gavrilovic. "Do we have to go to New York?"

"No," Ye said. "He's in the Basking Ridge location." Now I'd worked in the Basking Ridge area for the past 25 years give or take a couple months. One would think I would have noticed a Sloan Kettering facility somewhere.

Later that evening while Sally slept, the dogs keeping her company on the bed upstairs, I had reached my first point of medical surrender and had a quick conversation with whatever was looking after us.

"Look, this is all up to you. I'm putting all the control in your hands, win lose or draw, you're in charge."

It wasn't the last time I had this conversation, but realizing the path we traveled thus far, a path that brought us to Dr. Ye, something I had no hand in planning, it slowly dawned on me that letting "the power" do its job just might be the way to go.

Dr. Igor Gavrilovic is one of those guys that just looks smart. An oval face with studious, functional glasses, stocky build, wavy thick dark hair, and eyes that express the knowledge that his brain is constantly clattering away. Like Ye, he was honest and straightforward while being compassionate and, also like Ye, he confirmed what was going on in Sally's head.

Dr. G went straight to Chapter Two, Page 25 in the How to Be a Neurologist handbook, the section on Patient Examination. Every neurologist we encountered danced through the same set of instructions. The patients were given three things to remember and told that they will have to repeat them later. Inevitably, these three things involved a colored object, a place or number and a state or animal. I figured it was like a secret handshake or something that they all chuckled about at their neurological conventions.

"The three things I want you to remember are red rooster, 35, and Rhode Island. Can you say them back to me?"

Sally repeated them.

Dr. G continued. "What day of the week is it?" "Month?" "Year?" "Where are we"? "Who is vice-president?" [2]

Sally scored about 75% on her answers, the Veep and the month stumping her.

"Now," he said, "spell 'world' backwards." [3]

Sally sat silently trying to think it through, but then so was I. I had to spell it forwards in my mind. "D." She paused. I was in the habit of answering everything else for her lately so biting my tongue through the testing became a tough challenge.

She continued. "R". "O". "L". "W".

Dr. G smiled. "Okay. That's fine."

I learned I'm way too OCD to be a doctor; my instinct was geared toward making sure she got it right. Somehow I kept my mouth shut… for a change.

Then came all the physical tests: walking a straight line, tests for coordination, peripheral vision, and limb weakness.

Then after all that, Dr. G. said, "What are the three things I asked you to remember?"

Sally stared at him, trying to break through the sludge in her brain.

---

2 This one irks me because I'm guessing 50% of the population wouldn't know who the Veep was even without brain lymphoma.

3 Seeing "world" written here makes it easy to spell backwards. Try doing it sometime out of the blue without it printed in front of you.

"One was a state," Dr. G. prompted.

"Rhode Island."

"Good."

Following another bit of silence Sally said, "Thirty-five." I was impressed. That was the one I couldn't remember.

"Great. And the third one?"

Sally's blank stare attested to her complete incomprehension; she was mentally lost in reciting even a small scrap of an answer.

"A color….and an animal…" Dr G. said. Still nothing. "Red…"

"Rooster," Sally chimed in.

I stopped chomping my tongue and gave myself an invisible pat on the back for maintaining silence.

Once the examination was completed, Dr. G started speaking in a different language. Ridiculously long drug names ending in "ate" or "ine,' phrases such as "seven treatments every other week," "four to five days in-patient," "we can knock this out completely."

While I was trying to decipher all this, Sally reiterated her question of primary importance. "Will I be able to keep my hair?"

I told you it was a big deal.

Dr. G. stated that it was possible very little hair loss would occur with the chemical stew they had concocted.

"And all this will be done here in Basking Ridge?" I asked.

"No, it has to be done in New York because of the need for in-patient care. Everything here is out-patient."

Crap.

I was not thrilled with the prospect of going to Manhattan. The city never represented a place of safety; all I ever knew about it is what the media fed me during the sixties and seventies. Those fears still gnawed at me even though the city had become somewhat safer over the years and, theoretically, I had matured.

In addition, my NYC hospital experiences to date were un-nerving and left me quite unimpressed with the dreary atmosphere of the facilities I visited. As if the stress of what Sally had endured thus far and what I imagined had yet to face wasn't enough, adding regular trips to Manhattan was like pouring gasoline on my stress level which was already a raging inferno.

We left Dr. G's office with enough informational paperwork to rival the Tolkien Trilogy and the knowledge that if they could find a bed at the New York facility, he wanted to start ASAP. The current census at the hospital was 110%. Busy place.

Once again, we stared into the abyss of the unknown -- the single worst place to be no matter what stage of the journey. Minutes are hours long and the days a blur of low-grade anxiety.

I sat in my office on the second floor of the house, watching the long shadows of the approaching winter play across the neighboring houses and leafless trees. I tried to stay as far out of my brain as I could. All I could do was rely on the force that brought us this far to keep us safe for the mystery that laid ahead.

What gives me peace in my life:

_____
_____
_____
_____
_____
_____
_____
_____
_____
_____
_____
_____

What action that gives me peace can I make a routine:

_____
_____
_____
_____
_____
_____

Notes:

Caregiver Tip #8

You are not alone.
Caregiving is a team sport. Take advantage of everyone who comes into your inner circle.

This is your new mantra:

ASK FOR HELP

The only person who expects you to take on all the caregiver burdens by yourself is....

YOU

Lots of people ask, "What can I do?" The typical caregiver knee-jerk reaction is "nothing". In order to change "nothing" into something concrete, make a list of all the things you have on your plate. Assign half of them to other people. You will be surprised how quickly people will jump at the chance to do something...anything. The hardest aspect of being a caregiver is asking for help. *Do it anyway.*

News Headlines...

Monday November 24th, 2014:

- Best rap hip/hop album at Sunday's American Music Awards Ceremony was won by Australian Iggy Azalea.

- The smoldering kindling of Ferguson, MO exploded as officials delayed announcing the Grand Jury decision of the Darrell Wilson/Michael Brown case until after the sun had set.

- A California tour bus tried to place an order at Denny's by taking a pass on the drive-thru window and driving directly into the restaurant's kitchen.

- In Cleveland, a twelve-year-old BB gun toting idiot was having a good old time pointing his weapon at seniors in a recreation center. When asked by police to put his hands up, he chose instead to reach for his gun. He'll never get any older.

Sally and I were unaware of the day's lunacy while we waited for a call from Sloan Kettering with news of a vacancy. Whatever was happening in the rest of the world was far beyond our consideration. This was the day Dr. G told us to be ready to head for the city and start chemotherapy, assuming the hospital census dropped below 110% and there was a bed for us. In the meantime, Sally remained downstairs glued to the TV, and I doodled around on the internet in my upstairs office. At this point the reality of cancer still remained outside the safety of being entombed in the four walls of our house. Denial was a beautiful thing.

Everything that had happened in the journey thus far - changing doctors in the 11th hour, moving from one house to another that put us in a neighborhood close to where we originally lived, even Sally getting passout drunk on one drink – none of it was on our life radar, but because we were able to trust the calm voices speaking to us, all of these things brought us to a place where we needed to be. I had no doubts that we were in the right hands to get the care Sally needed.

Even more critical was being close enough to take advantage of the support we needed to make it all happen, particularly with the treatment schedule we faced, traveling to New York City every other week for eight treatments, each a three-to-five day, in-patient experience. Our daughter Beth and Sally's sister Katie were within a 15-minute drive of our new house and gladly agreed to look after our babies; the two dogs over-wrought with separation anxiety when Mom and Dad disappeared, but at least they remained in their home as opposed to the tension convention a trip to the kennel would bring every ten days. That and the money Kate and Beth saved us was significant. They worked out a coverage schedule, including spending nights in our house to make sure the dogs were taken care of in the morning. Had we ended up moving into the termite trap we contracted for and walked away from, this arrangement would not have been possible. Big red check mark on the gratitude list and yet another reason convincing us that we were where we were for a specific reason.

Lunch was finished and I was busy staring out my home office window, open to the balmy Thanksgiving week weather, just trying to breathe. I felt myself unwind…just a fraction.

Then the phone rang. A bed was waiting. Room 715A.

Sally was engrossed in story hour; the daily ritual between twelve and one in the afternoon when life comes to a screeching halt at the Cooper household, and we become immersed in the lives of Nicole, Zander, Brady, Mel, Serena[1]…"Like sand through an hourglass, so are the Days of Our Lives…"

As I walked into the den, I sat in front of Sally, took her hand, and said, "They have a room. Are you ready?"

That moment punched a Hulk-sized hole in the denial. Tears sprang from Sally's eyes. I just held her.

"We can do this," I said. "We'll do it together." I said that to convince myself as much as Sally.

Facing the task of physically leaving the house took the wind out of both our sails, so we took a few seconds to silently say goodbye to life as we knew it.

---

1 Oh, dear God, I know these people's names.

Of the 52 weeks of the year that this first visit could have taken place, the week it did was the second to last choice on the list. What were the odds it would land on Thanksgiving week?

We knew this first visit was going to last five to seven days. Spending Thanksgiving in the hospital ranked right up there with enduring a root canal without Novocaine and having my eyelashes waxed.

With the windows open, the wind whipped through the car as we drove north on the New Jersey Turnpike past the industrial oil tanks, Newark Airport, and billboards aimed at amplifying religious guilt. Near the airport two incongruous signs, less than 30 yards apart, moved into view. The first touting an upcoming conference aimed at empowering women. The second reminding drivers to come to the New Jersey Conference Center for this weekend's grand opening of the XXX Adult World Trade Show.

"Well, that was well thought out," I said, in an attempt to ease the tension. Sally rewarded my efforts with a wan smile.

Surprisingly, the drive across Manhattan on 53rd, which was usually a jam-packed, bumper-car death race, was uncluttered. Landmarks such as Carnegie Hall on 8th Avenue and the 5th Avenue jewelry intersection ushered us toward the east side.

Having dutifully read the pre-treatment literature, we were prepared for the line of cars that trailed from the 66th Street entrance to the MSK parking garage and stretched around the corner cascading down York Avenue. I had never visited the east side of the city. The level of perceived threat looked low, the neighborhood a mix of residential and half a dozen different hospitals.

Time dragged as we inched forward, allowing my paranoia free-will to roam. The apartment buildings on 66th ran the gamut from newer white brick and chrome to the early 20th century chocolate brown row houses.

The three-car-width street itself looked okay; I saw no sign that gang warfare was about to erupt.

At one point a shiny BMW turned onto 66th and stopped next to the cars backed up at the garage entrance with the clear intention of cutting in. As if choreographed, every car simultaneously inched that much closer to the car in front of them, sending the universal "Fuck you if you think you are getting in here" message. The Beemer sat stubbornly waiting to be let in, which not only pissed everyone off who waited in line, but also blocked all remaining 66th street traffic from passing. Cabs loved this. If the wind changes direction, NYC cabdrivers lean on their horns. The automotive cacophony kicked in from the blocked motorists as the Beemer steadfastly refused all the gentle hints provided, until one of the garage attendants emerged from the depths and politely motioned for the car to get the hell out of the way, drive around the block and get in line like everybody else. As the car sped away, I was comforted that someone from the hospital stood up for those of us in queue.

We eventually nudged our way onto the ramp going into the garage and abandoned our car there once the attendant handed us a ticket and said, "How long will you be?"

"Friday or Saturday," I said.

A knowing flicker briefly crossed his face and as we walked away, he said, "Good luck.'

Walking further into the garage looked, from my vantage point on the ramp, as if we were walking into a multi-car pile-up. I led us out of the garage onto 66th and just started walking. I figured I had a 50-50 chance of walking in the correct direction.

Reaching 1st Avenue, I concluded lady luck was not on my side so we stopped a fresh-faced young man wearing a while lab coat, which had to mean he was medically connected in some way,[2] and asked for directions to the hospital entrance.

"Oh that's one street over, I think." he said, filling me with confidence.

We continued walking north on First Avenue, then, still not seeing anything like an entrance, we turned east onto 67th, right back down the hill to York Avenue.

A spark of memory clicked in: It's somewhere on York. Yes. York. We crossed York because there were some really nice-looking hospital buildings across the street, which turned out to be New York Presbyterian Hospital. Feeling like true tourists as we lugged our rolling suitcases around the East Side, I finally spotted the entrance – on the opposite side of York Avenue. Figured.

We started to cross back over York, but not before a young gentleman of the homeless variety started relating his sad tale to Sally, who had stopped to play captive audience and was gearing up to help this poor soul in any way she could; homeless people, lost animals – as a Libra, Sally wanted to help everyone. After explaining to the man that we were late for chemotherapy, and that Sally's communication capabilities were on the fritz, he backed off and I led Sally across York.

"Your own current sob story takes precedence over those of other folks for the time being," I said.

We finally arrived and took what would be the first of many steps into 1275 York Avenue.

Admissions? Bah. Who needs admissions! We went straight to room 715A, parked our butts, and waited. Most of the rooms are double occupancy but neither bed was occupied. Staff members walked by and gave us

---

2 Or he was part of a white lab coat cult – this was New York City after all

very odd looks, wondering who these crazy people were just hanging out in an empty room.

As hospital rooms go, this one was fairly bright and cheerful; white walls with large windows that allowed gobs of ambient light to shine through. I've been in other hospital rooms in Manhattan where bad lighting and prison porthole windows created a dim yellow haze, sort of like the Civil War triage scenes from Gone with the Wind.

We stood in what was to be our new home for the next five to seven days waiting for something to happen. My mind wandered to my sole experience with cancer nursing to date. Two days after my mother's cancer surgery, the nursing staff, who all looked like former defensive linemen for the Oakland Raiders, ignored the list of medications Mom was allergic to and administered a morphine-based pain killer, which for my mom, was not much different than giving her three or four hits of White Lightning. Once the hallucinations kicked in, they strapped her down to the hospital bed and let her ride through it. All this happened overnight so none of us knew about it until the next day.

Needless to say, I walked into MSK with a chip on my shoulder and my best suit of armor, daring anyone to make a wrong move.

"Mrs. Cooper? Hi. I'm Kristyn."

I snapped out of my revery to see a pixie with long brown hair and a sunshine smile who looked as if she would be at home on a West Coast beach sipping an umbrella drink.

"We're a bit chaotic today. Lots of patients being discharged with just as many new ones waiting to come in."

"You need rollerblades," I said.

"Oh, tell me about it," Kristyn said in her best Valley Girl smile, as she erased the small whiteboard near Sally's bed, drew a line horizontally across it, then wrote "AM" on the top half followed by "Kristyn" with a heart drawn next to it. We'd find out who belonged on the PM half later.

"Let me get you a hospital gown and all the other stuff you'll need. You can wear sweats underneath it if you want. Whatever works for you. I'll be back to check you out and go over the schedule."

Score one for the nurse community.

The rest of the day was a whirlwind of people. Kristyn getting Sally gowned up, comfortable in bed, a pic line inserted into her hand, food menus, bathrooms and general expectations.

Then the tornado whirled into the room.

"Hey! What's up? I'm Liz, Nurse Practitioner Extraordinaire."

She immediately started in with, "You will kick this with no problem. Happens all the time."

I kept looking for her pompoms and megaphone embroidered sweater. If it was possible to harness energy from someone's aura, we could lick any crisis on Liz's frenetic optimism alone. A full head shorter than Sally, Liz was a dark-haired, Irish fireball with piercing eyes. If she had sported a tattoo that read "no bullshit," I would not have been surprised.

Liz explained what was going to happen over the next few days. Another MRI, a PET scan, a bone marrow biopsy and a spinal tap, all so they could start chemo on Thursday – how's that for a Thanksgiving Dinner? Both Sally and I groaned at the spinal tap, relating our Philadelphia experience, the one similar to having a manicure with railroad spikes and a sledgehammer. A look of shock came over Liz's face.

"Seriously?" she said. "No. That's not right. We don't like them for telling you that. No, you'll be on your back for the day after the procedure and trust me, you'll be fine."

Even though it was day one, there was a spark inside me, a slowly calming realization that Sally was going to be taken care of by a nursing staff that was the direct opposite of my mom's experience. I started relaxing, feeling that I did not have to be on watch 24/7 to make sure Sally's treatment wasn't half-assed.

Kristyn returned, asking background questions, symptoms, timing etc. Sally would say two or three words then look at me as if to say, "I could use some help here." So I stepped in as her mouthpiece, giving Kristyn all the backstory that got us to Sloan and what was going on in Sally's world, the MS saga, the hideous spinal tap experience. Even if Sally could remember it all, putting the story to words was still an impossible task.

"One important question -- is there somewhere I can sleep?" I asked Kristyn.

"I'll get a sleeper chair for you. They can be tough to find because we don't have a lot of them, but I will track one down." She was so matter of fact and sure about everything. If I had asked her to find a lisping blue and green house cat, Kristyn would have smiled and said, "Sure, no problem." And probably would have found one. I liked her more and more.

An array of white and pink jacketed medical-types popped in the room every ten minutes, or so it seemed, to take Sally's temperature, blood pressure, urine samples, and blood samples. They performed mini checkups on Sally's optic reactions, looked for sores in her mouth, and to see if any new symptoms arose; not a short process as their massive symptom menu was longer than any New Jersey diner menu. Sally and I went through our explanatory song and dance for each new face that arrived.

We sat in the room watching Food Network, which had become the de facto channel (except for the daily story hour, of course), when in walked a mountain, bulging out of a royal blue hospital shirt with a smile a mile wide and pushing a wheelchair.

"Mrs. Cooper," which, with the heavy island accent, sounded more like "Mz. Koopah." "I'm David. Ready to take a ride?" David was there to take Sally for her MRI and PET scan. "Is dis your other half?" he said pointing at me and offering a beefy hand. "You sit tight, Pop, and we have her back in no time." To Sally he said, "I brought your limo." Sally had yet to be connected to an IV drip so the bed could stay and the wheelchair limo was sufficient transportation.

As they both waved at me rolling down the hall, I was jolted by the thought that the purpose of the scans and taps and biopsies was to ascertain if there were any additional cancer growths in Sally's body. That thought never entered my mind, but now it put a knot in my gut, imagining what other traumas Sally would have to endure if the junk in her brain was not the only issue.

To kill some time, I performed a little online research and read that it was common for brain lymphoma to be a secondary cancer, caused by the spreading of another variant in the body.

The more I read, the more frightened I became, and the more I started convincing myself that the existing lymphoma was only the tip of the iceberg. Complicated chemo and radiation scenarios danced in my head, each episode more disastrous than the next. (*See Caregiver Tip #3 concerning internet usage - Learn from my mistakes!*)

I finally just turned off my phone and ventured out into the corridor to get the lay of the land, finding where a few minor things were, like water, ice, a Coke machine and a bathroom I could use. There were two bathrooms in the hallway, each the size of a standard chimney flue. One was for guests, and one was marked Staff Only. This was going to be interesting.

Back in 715A, I glanced at the pile of literature thrown at incoming patients and saw…a menu. A menu? This is a hospital. In my experience, hospital food choices were completed by circling items on a three by five sheet, and then being served something inedible at some random future point.

Near dinner time, Sally read off some of the items. "Chicken stir fry, short ribs…" then trailed off into the inability to speak further…

She handed me the menu and I continued reading, "Pizza, burgers, soup. Oh, cool; ice cream." Sally's eyes lit up at that. "How about this, chicken stir fry, some French fries, a Diet Coke and some vanilla ice cream."

"Yeah," she said with a smile. I called the magic food service number and got an actual person.

I placed the order, curious to see if the final product measured up to the process.

Some time later, a waiter arrived. At least I assumed so based on his attire; black slacks, pressed white shirt and black vest. My first thought was that he was visiting someone while on a break from one of the local restaurants.

"Mrs. Cooper?" he said with a hint of a Spanish accent. Sally nodded in acknowledgement. He turned back to the hallway then brought in a tray of covered dishes and all the goodies we had ordered from the food service.

"My name is Marco. Please let me know if you need anything. Enjoy." He had a balding Charlie Brown face with just a hint of hesitation, as if double checking himself to make sure he didn't do anything wrong.

"Thank you," Sally said, and he left the room with a smile.

To both our amazement the food was not only hot, a real hospital rarity, but also pretty damn tasty.

"If it weren't for the cancer, this would be a nice place to hang out," I said

While Sally was eating, an ungodly scraping noise sounded from the hallway, faint at first, but growing louder as it headed in the direction of our room. Before I could get up to look, a blue vinyl beast with oak arms turned the corner into our room with impish little Kristyn pushing its back as if herding it into a pen.

"Found one," she said triumphantly, standing next to the sleeper chair as if she had just bagged it on an African veldt. It looked like a normal chair on steroids, was hideously uncomfortable to sit in, but once I figured out how the contraption unfolded into a cot-like bed, I was grateful to have it.

Near seven that night, Kristyn walked in, 12-hour shift exhaustion showing on her face, accompanied by another young woman, in the nurse garb of white pants, shirt and blue zip-up sweatshirt - they were all dressed as if heading for a track meet - which isn't far off from accurate in the physical sense.

"This is Alexa," Kristyn said. "She's on duty overnight." Alexa stood a foot taller than Kristyn, brown hair falling across her shoulders, with the same award winning-smile as Kristyn.[3]

There was a spark of discomfort inside me, fueled by the preposterous thought of wanting Kristyn to stay for the duration. Did we really have to change nurses? I was just getting comfortable. The thought of Kristyn working 24 hours was immaterial.

Alexa arrived later to give Sally the once over, asking the same series of questions with me providing the backstory. She had the same warm demeanor as Kristyn.

---

[3] I guess the image of matronly, cranky grandmother types as nurses is part of a bygone era. All these young women were bright, personable and complete knockouts.

I spent the first night lying in my sleeper chair wide awake and counting the acoustic tile holes, which gazed back down at me like a million black stars. What in God's name was I doing in a hospital in New York City lying on a piece of furniture that transformed into Optimus Prime?

From out of nowhere, a voice started needling me that I should keep some sort of journal, which is unusual for me. I'm a writer but keeping a diary/journal on a daily basis is not something at which I've ever succeeded.

It occurred to me that chronicling this journey in some fashion might serve two purposes:

- **Keep me occupied – thus not losing my mind.**
- **Keep everyone else informed of what was happening.**

Okay three purposes.

- **Ensuring we maintained a sense of humor and a positive perspective.**

"Fringe Observations" felt like a good title for the ongoing Facebook journal as that was exactly where I stood, on the fringe, observing every person, place and thing connected with this odyssey.

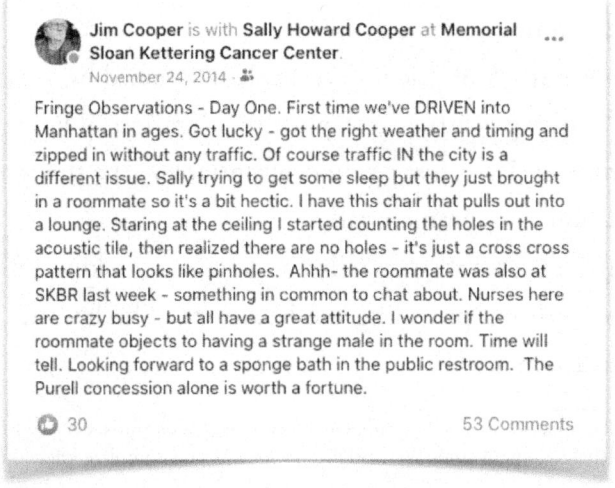

> Jim Cooper is with Sally Howard Cooper at Memorial Sloan Kettering Cancer Center.
> November 24, 2014
>
> Fringe Observations - Day One. First time we've DRIVEN into Manhattan in ages. Got lucky - got the right weather and timing and zipped in without any traffic. Of course traffic IN the city is a different issue. Sally trying to get some sleep but they just brought in a roommate so it's a bit hectic. I have this chair that pulls out into a lounge. Staring at the ceiling I started counting the holes in the acoustic tile, then realized there are no holes - it's just a cross cross pattern that looks like pinholes. Ahhh- the roommate was also at SKBR last week - something in common to chat about. Nurses here are crazy busy - but all have a great attitude. I wonder if the roommate objects to having a strange male in the room. Time will tell. Looking forward to a sponge bath in the public restroom. The Purell concession alone is worth a fortune.
>
> 30   53 Comments

As first days go, I was feeling only mildly unsettled, as opposed to the stomach-churning, pre-hospital insanity. There was still much to come our way, I thought. Tuesday was spinal tap day, Wednesday, the bone marrow biopsy and first dose of chemo and then Thursday, a Thanksgiving portion of "the big gun," the high-dose chemo. Sally was taking it all in stride. She had adopted the attitude of turning everything over to MSK and hanging on for the ride. Cautious optimism remained my state of mind; I still felt on duty, walking the parapets in preparation for the oncoming attack.

Marco had become our friend very quickly, I think primarily because we remembered his name whenever we saw him. One afternoon I pulled him aside and complimented him on the job he was doing. You'd be surprised how far that can go in a service industry, especially one where people bitch and moan at the drop of a fork. Marco told me that he would get anything that we wanted, even if it wasn't on the menu.

It is impossible to live in a bisected ten by fifteen-foot room with another person and not figure out their medical story, even if the roommates don't verbally connect. By day two Sally and her late arriving roomie, Kathie[4], were chatting through the overgrown shower curtain separating the room. This was Kathie's third time around, having beat breast and lung cancer. Now it had leached into her spine, and she had just spent a week at the surgical center having a portion of her spine repaired. I had trouble digesting that -- repairing a spine? The more I learned what medical science was achieving in this battle, the more I was astounded.

That morning, our nurse of the day, Jasmine, a moon-faced sweetheart with skin the color of caramel apples and massive glasses over sparkling dark eyes, came into the room dressed in the standard white pants, shirt and blue zip-up hoodie.

---

4 Name changed out of respect for privacy and fear the HIPPA stormtroopers will come get me.

Name changed out of respect for privacy and fear the HIPPA stormtroopers will come get me. "Hey guys'" she said, "Just wanted to let you know the results of the MRI and the PET scan were negative. They didn't find anything."

We both breathed a sigh of relief.

Liz bounced into the room behind Jasmine to lend support for the test of the day, the second spinal tap. "You'll be fine. We do these all the time. You'll be on your back the rest of the day, but you'll breeze through it."

An odd thought popped in my head. "Why can't you use the results from the first spinal tap?" I asked.

"The first spinal tap tested only for MS symptoms. None of the cancer tests were conducted on the first draw of spinal fluid," Liz said.

"Pardon me, but if lymphoma is a distinct possibility, I'd have thought testing for both, or any possibilities, at the same time made more sense."

Just one more item proving that leaving Philadelphia General was a positive move. On the downside, here was another test that could possibly find other, and in my mind more serious cancer cells, because we were delving into spinal fluid. My stress level approached off-the-meter Richter scale proportions.

David came rolling into the room. "They ready for you, Miz Cooper." Instead of a wheelchair, Sally's bed provided the transportation this time; they were serious about keeping her on her back which was just fine with me.

Sally's tolerance for immobility ranks with… well, let's be honest; she has none. So when David piloted her back into the room, I was prepared to spend the day battling to keep her still.

"How'd it go?" I asked.

"Fine. They just numbed me up and did their thing."

"And now you're going to remain flat on your back for eight hours, right?"

Her answer surprised me. "Absolutely. I'm not going through that again."

Obviously, this was not the hospital's first rodeo as the swivel arm holding the TV protruding from the wall made adjusting the TV for someone flat on their back a no-brainer. Sally opted for a liquid lunch - not the good kind unfortunately - out of convenience and to avoid me making a half-assed attempt at feeding her and spilling food all over her and the bed.

By mid-afternoon, one of the biggest hurdles in this process reared its torpid head: **BOREDOM**

Aside from ensuring Sally was in good shape I needed to find stuff to occupy my downtime. I don't have Sally's patience for TV watching; after an hour or so glued to the mindless blather of daytime TV, I'm ready to stick my tongue in a light socket. I had no issue, however, cruising the internet until my eyes bled.

Upon opening Facebook I was stunned to find over 80 comments and/or likes to the first cancer post from the previous night, with more than 25 percent from our Westfield High Class of '74. I was floored. I showed it to Sally and as she scrolled through the comments, the tears flowed harder and harder.

"I don't get it," she kept saying. "Who am I anyway?" She couldn't fathom the impact she had on so many people.

By late afternoon, Jasmine reappeared and raised the head of Sally's bed about ten degrees.

"I want to check you out," she said. "Your spinal tap results were negative, but we still have to go through the routine."

"That was fast," I said, genuinely surprised. We waited two weeks to get spinal tap results from Philly General; MSK took less than six hours.

Wednesday morning, Shirley, Sally's assigned nurse that day, suggested[5] Sally get her ass out of bed and walk around. Our reaction was guarded, bordering on terror. The morning passed, however, with no repercussions. It's amazing what medical competency can achieve. Shirley, the most soft spoken of the nurses but with broad-faced smile that lit up the room, came in to check on her patient. Even though Shirley was reserved, almost shy, I had the feeling that crossing her would be a mistake. I went through our backstory, again, bringing Shirley up to speed.

After she left, I said to Sally, "I need to record the whole story and just play it for each new doctor or nurse who comes in. I feel like a broken record saying the same thing over and over."

That afternoon two lads in white lab coats sauntered into Sally's room, announcing they were going to perform the bone marrow biopsy.

"Right here?" I said as my brain produced horror film scenarios about the pain involved in the procedure, having heard nightmarish tales about bone marrow tests. I wasn't sure I could listen to Sally screaming in pain while these guys administered a Han Solo type torture. Sterility concerns placed a distant, but still important, second.

"Mr. Cooper," said the lab coat in charge, "we need you to leave the room."

It's very Ward Cleaver of me, but I do jump into the protector role when any possibility of physical pain comes near those I love. My discomfort doubles when the pain comes in the name of science, and there is absolutely nothing I can do about it. I thought about challenging him on

---

5 Kind of like the "suggestions" troops received from General Patton.

this request; it certainly wasn't for sterility reasons and just what the actual hell were they going to do to Sally?

I kept forgetting, however, that my official status on the floor was "visitor," which knocked my willingness to cause a scene down a few pegs. When "a visitor" is thrown out of a hospital room at a medical person's request, there are only two things to do. One, try not to make other patients feel like they are on display as you loiter aimlessly in the hallway past their rooms or, two, go to the cafeteria for a five dollar cup of coffee.

The nurse's station, a large bullpen of desks and computers sequestered behind glass decorated with signs and Thanksgiving cutouts, more to block the view of probing eyes than for atmosphere, was directly across from Sally's room. Taking two steps out of the room put me at the nurse's station window, staring in with a face pathetic enough to rival Oliver Twist begging for more gruel. I caught Shirley's eye, and she stopped what she was doing and popped out of the door.

"Everything okay?" she asked.

"I think so. They kicked me out while they do the bone marrow biopsy."

"Oh. Okay," she said and went back to her computer, which struck me as odd. Why wasn't she flying into hysterics and shooting me up with Darvon? "What about some tranquilization for the caregivers, huh?" I wanted to scream.[6]

Other than interrupting the nursing staff, keeping them from doing their work and generally making a nuisance of myself, I wasn't sure what else I could do at that moment other than wander the hallways. As I turned the corner coming down the home stretch of my first lap around the floor, I was more than a bit surprised to see the lab coats exiting room

---

6 One night when Kristyn checked up on Sally, asking if she needed an Ativan or something to settle her down, I chimed in that I could use a couple but was told with that dazzling smile that the drugs were for patients only. Damn.

715. I hurried back in, expecting to see Sally flat on her back, white as a ghost sporting a sickly death mask from her horrible experience.

Instead, I saw her sitting up in bed, the Food Network still flashing on the TV and sipping water from a pitcher.

"Hi," I said. Master of the quick wit that I am.

"Hey," she replied.

"So how was it?"

I received the usual response. "Fine. No problem. They just numbed me up, did their thing and left. Didn't hurt at all."

I wanted to run out of the room and hug everyone on staff. One of these days I'll let go of all the medical nightmare scenarios I create. It never occurred to me to ask anyone -- nurses, doctors, Marco, the cleaning staff -- what I should have expected during the biopsy procedure. That would have made far too much sense.

Okay. Testing is out of the way. Now the fun can begin.

The last time we were in Manhattan on Thanksgiving Day[7] was 2007 on a balmy, 60-degree day, a perfect time for a family excursion into the city to see the Thanksgiving Day parade in person. Seven Thanksgivings later, temperatures were in the twenties and since no one was about to let us go traipsing out of the hospital bound for Macy's on Eighth Avenue, we opted to watch the parade on TV.

I said to Sally, "It would be cool if they re-routed the parade to York Avenue so all the patients, especially the kids, could watch from their hospital room windows."

---

[7] Ever notice that many Thanksgiving illustrations show a cartoon turkey, wearing a chef's hat and grinning from ear to ear? That's like Jesus serving cocktails to the Romans on Good Friday…It still felt odd knowing the floats, balloons and pseudo-celebs were a mere seven avenues to the west of us, kind of like watching a Yankee home game while sitting in a bar across from the stadium.

"That would be nice," she said with a smirk.

"I'll have to write Mayor de Blasio a heartfelt letter."

"Good luck with that," she said, seriously and not reacting to my attempt at humor.

"What's the matter?"

She shrugged and didn't respond. I had no doubts at all about what was going on in her head.

"Hey," I said, curling on the end of the bed so we were face to face. "Yeah, it's Thanksgiving and you'd rather be at Katie's house with everyone, right?"

She looked up at the TV instead of me; I saw her eyes start welling up. Family was everything to Sally, and being separated from siblings, kids and grandkids on a family holiday drove red hot skewers into her core.

I said, "We'll call later and talk to them once they've gathered at Katie's. I know it's not the same, but this is where we need to be right now."

"I know," she said quietly, head down. "Doesn't make it easier."

We spent the day napping, eating a half-decent Thanksgiving dinner that Sloan had whipped up, and decided we felt sorrier for the hospital staff who got tagged with the holiday shift than we should for ourselves. The level of care remained constant, however, without any griping -- in front of the patients anyway. If it were me on call, I'd have bitched to anyone who would listen.

Just after dinner, with Sally still a little blue, I followed up on my promise and placed a FaceTime call to the family. Katie answered and I sat next to Sally on the bed so we both could peer into the Thanksgiving world some 60 miles away.

Everyone was gathered around the dinner table although it appeared the main course had been inhaled, everyone leaning back in their chairs in gluttonous repose. Stephen and Beth sat on one side of the table, Katie and her husband John's friends Mike and Laura sat on the other side. All the younger kids were off playing video games or glued to the TV.

Even though Sally was glassy-eyed through the whole conversation, making her a part of the day and being able to see her kids, made up for a small portion of not being able to attend in person.

Spending Thanksgiving in Chez Sloan was one thing, but Christmas was around the corner; how would I cope with the added frenzy of shopping, decorating, and shoveling (God forbid), not to mention the usual family get togethers?

I put those questions aside momentarily as we faced the immediate concern: The Chemo Big Gun.

The image I had of "chemo" was something between Colin Clive as Dr. Frankenstein re-animating the monster and Hollywood 1950s B-Movie depictions of radiation exposure. Needless to say, my vision was overly dramatic and confused, throwing chemo and radiation into the same medically-evil canoe. Did I ask anyone? Of course not.

Around ten that night, I became curious why the "big gun" round of chemo had not started yet. We were both shagged out, and it was already an hour past Sally's usual crash time.

Finally, a new bag was hung on Sally's IV stand and plugged into her feed.

"This is an anti-nausea drug," the nurse explained. "It helps counter any reactions you may have to the chemo."

It wasn't until 11 that night that another yellow-coated nurse strode into the room.

"Mrs. Cooper? I'm Mary and I'll be administering your chemo," she said exuding an authoritative air. In comparison to the 20-somethings in charge of the floor, Mary was an older woman of at least 30, blonde, and appeared to have trouble smiling; she was all business. In her hands was a plastic IV bag containing a yellow liquid that looked as if it had already been through someone.

Seeing that all the chemo nurses were dressed as if preparing for cleanup duties at Chernobyl, I began to feel somewhat vulnerable sitting there in just jeans and a t-shirt. Should I have some sort of protective shield or something? It's like getting X-rays at the dentist when they leave the room before the zap you. Excuse me, but if this machine will make you glow in the dark and turn your sperm into mutations, what the hell is it doing to me, especially pressed up against my face? I always expect skin to peel off in pink and red chunks a la Poltergeist.

After Mary finished double verifying that they were administering the proper dosage of the right drug to the right patient, she explained in layman's terms exactly what this stuff they were sticking in Sally's body would do, how the drug operates at a cellular level, and the scientific theory of the outcome. I was fascinated with her explanation and happy she took the time to explain it all. More importantly, I felt a sense of empowerment. Most of this journey is spent blindly groping through a dark basement, reaching out in hopes of finding a light switch before stepping on a nail or smashing a toe into any immovable object. With a deeper understanding of the intricacies of chemotherapy, my fear of the process decreased from the Pennywise monster I had imagined, into something that made sense, something I could wrap my head around.

"This is why you have to be monitored for three or four days after treatment," Mary said. "We have to ensure you've flushed out a sufficient amount of the drug so it's no longer lethal to the organs in your body. You will get blood drawn every day to check the level of this chemo drug remaining in your system. Once it gets to or below a specific count, they will release you. It usually takes two or three days."

While the drug dripped into Sally's veins, she drifted off to sleep and I looked online for the name of the drug and started reading about the down-and-dirty science of it, which was not unlike reading Christmas Eve toy assembly instructions written in a code requiring Little Orphan Annie's secret decoder pin:

"This molecule binds with the 4th nitrogen strain of the ZX6-23stp DNA chain..."

Holy crap! Thank God someone understood all that.

Every science teacher who had tolerated me from grade school through college will attest to the fact that my science skills were as nimble as a one-legged frog leaping out of a puddle of 10w-30 Quaker State motor oil. It was never my strong suit. Come to think of it neither was history. Nor English. Nor social studies. I excelled at study hall.

So I gave a silent shout-out to every science teacher I ever had: Mr. Kashuba, Mr. Fine, Ms. Kresch, Mr. Elder, Mrs. Foster, and Dr. McGrath. Thankfully, you ignited the scientific spark in other kids who went on to become the creators of the drugs that have kept Sally and thousands of other cancer patients alive.

The drip finished up around one in the morning. I was wide awake and on-watch. When does the chaos kick in, I thought. Here I was waiting for Sally to sprout a second head or go into snake wiggling, bible-thumping seizures and convulsions. At a minimum to have all her hair instantly drop off her head like a collapsing house of cards. Given my penchant for producing nightmare medical scenarios, the reality was anti-climactic. Which was just fine; don't get me wrong.

By two in the morning the infusions were done and Sally was out cold. However, my nightly Sisyphean sleep attempt was compounded by the niggling voice in my head reminding me that the bone marrow biopsy results were still unknown.

I became self-sufficient in finding amusing distractions when sleep remained elusive. After strolling around the silent, empty corridors for awhile, I found an empty chair in the hallway, made myself comfortable, and started watching an old Dean Martin Roast on YouTube[8], where a nearly unrecognizable, American-Top-40 Casey Kasem made up as Adolph Hitler was masquerading as roastee Don Rickles joke writer. I didn't think of it in terms of necessary caregiver escapism - that wouldn't hit home until the next day.

However, for the moment, I breathed easier, grateful the day was over and the experience uneventful.

---

8 It remains inconceivable to me that I sat in a silent hospital hallway at two in the morning with a high resolution TV screen the size of a business card and watched Hollywood legends on a Dean Martin Roast make fun of Don Rickles. Especially to those of us old enough to remember getting out of the chair to change the channel and pray the rabbit ears could lock on to some watchable signal on channels 2, 4, 5, 7, 9, or 11. PBS/13 was an option but only if all other resources were exhausted and only if Sesame Street was on.

My Caregiver support team:

Notes:

Make self-care a priority
Pay attention to your own needs

Caregiver Tip #9

Get enough sleep, eat healthy foods, take a nap, take a walk...do whatever you can to give yourself downtime, even when feelings of guilt arise - which they will. Not only are you permitted to take breaks, it's a requirement. If the caregiver gets sick....

On Friday morning, Kristyn was back on duty and when she came in, I made a valiant effort at removing the web from my sleep-deprived face and asked, "Have we heard anything back from the bone marrow biopsy?"

"Let me find out for you," she said, which meant she would find out after she and Sally chatted for ten or fifteen minutes, three of which were medical and the rest about our kids and Kristyn's upcoming wedding. Outside the leafless trees swayed under a grey sky. The Indian summer that ushered us into the hospital had made room for the onset of impending winter. Street activity looked sparse; the east side of Manhattan is not the Mecca of Black Friday retail insanity and the few people scurrying about were bundled up in recently unpacked down jackets, hats and scarves.

"How are you feeling?" I asked Sally.

"I'm fine. I keep waiting for something bad to happen but so far nothing."

"Works for me." I called room service for Sally and trundled to the cafeteria hoping to grab some eggs and sausage for myself, but as we had slept in, the pickings were slim - possibly due to the later hour or possibly from post-Thanksgiving hangovers. Suddenly, I heard a voice beckoning me: "Goooo toooo the Coffee Shop."

Upon entering I was greeted by the usual hospital-coffee-shop inventory: get well cards, word search books, flowers, floating get well balloons, the entire bear family from Goldilocks - in stuffed form - and, of course, coffee. Stacked next to the urns was an assortment of pre-packaged oatmeal-in-a-cup. Going with the cinnamon apple flavor (in my mind, the maple brown sugar version sort of defeats any nutritious benefits of the oatmeal), I got in the checkout line and there...there in a small rack sitting atop the shelf over the freezer with Klondike Bars and Chipwiches, were individually wrapped slabs of heaven. Coffee cake. But not just "coffee cake." I'm talking two-inch-thick slices that were half yellow cake, and half cinnamon crumble topping with the merest dusting of powdered sugar. I surrendered all free will and watched my arm automatically grab a cellophane wrapped piece.

"These are wonderful. They are made with real butter," said the checkout lady who resembled Mrs. Claus. As if I needed any further incentive to contribute to the cause of my impending coronary. Back in the room I shared my treasure with Sally, even though my instinct was to go all Golom-like and crouch in the corner, "I'll protect you, Precious."

Sally was not a junk food eater, so I had held out gluttonous hope that I could devour the slab of cake on my own. "Want some?" I offered.

"Sure."

Damn. We each took a bite.

"Oh wow," Sally said.

"Holy crap."

"This is outrageous," she said breaking off another hunk. "From the cafeteria?"

"Coffee shop," I said with a mouthful as powdered sugar flew off my lips.

"Cooper, this is excellent." I was shocked. When it comes to sweets, Sally's focus is ice cream. Period. Cake, pie, chocolate, cookies...none of it turned her on in any way.

While we languished in our sugar coma, Kristyn bopped into the room.

"The bone marrow biopsy was clear," she said with a wide grin, knowing this was great news. The ability to breate returned. I spent the morning sending silent "thank yous" in gratitude to whatever force was out there.

Chef Anne Burrell was showing us what to do with Thanksgiving leftovers on TV. Sally and I half-dozed; the week's stress of procedures and drugs slowly dissipating. Now, it was just a waiting game, hoping Sally would flush the chemo out of her system quickly.

Suddenly, a crowd of people burst into the room. I wasn't sure if I was asleep or not, but I recognized all of the faces - and it was people dressed normally in street clothes, not hospital pinks, whites and blues.

"Oh my God," Sally and I said in unison as Katie, Beth, Sally's brother Chris and her Aunt Betsy and Uncle Warren surprised us with a visit. Warren and Betsy lived in Southeastern Pennsylvania, and Chris lived a stone's throw from the Cape May, New Jersey ferry so it took effort to make the trek into the city. Sally noticeably brightened up with all the company, providing some direct family interaction after a trying Thanksgiving Day.

Even with all the extra people being close to Sally, I lurked on the outskirts of the group keeping an eye of the activity around her. The thought of walking away and letting someone maintain a watch on Sally produced feelings of fear. And guilt. It was, after all, my job to be the eyes, ears and brains of Sally's treatment, and if something were to happen and I wasn't there, it would, somehow, be my fault.

Ten minutes into the visit, Warren, as my surrogate father, got in my face and said, "Come on. We're taking you out to lunch. You need a break."

I did? My whole body tightened. Is that allowed, I thought. I felt like a soldier deserting his post. I'm not supposed to show any weakness or lapses in caregiving coverage.

Katie and Beth were going to stay with Sally while Warren, Betsy, Chris and I headed out into the city. My natural instinct was hesitation, but it was four against one and with my in-laws, it's better to acquiesce and admit defeat than maintain a weakened position.

In my stupor I followed Warren, Betsy and Chris to a spiffy Italian place on Lexington Avenue that used real plates and silver knives and forks instead of plastic utensils and Styrofoam clamshell boxes. I kept looking, in vain, for the cafeteria trays. As we sat in a softly lit dining room, I felt something at my core give way. I felt the good, nutritious food battle the onslaught of sugar I had subjected my body to earlier in the day. A flood of calm, letting go of the sentinel that had been on watch twenty-four seven for the previous five days. Like pressing a tautly wound joy-buzzer, my muscles became pliable once again, I could swivel my head in an arc greater than 20 degrees. This was a huge lesson for me as a caretaker. I needed to start paying attention to what I was thinking, feeling, eating and doing or else I could easily keep moving at a hundred miles an hour without ever seeing the fast-approaching brick wall.

It took some effort at first, but over the course of Sally's treatment, I found ways to make sure I got the rest, decompression and nurturing I needed to keep going. It wasn't until late in the game I discovered that even with all that I did, it wasn't nearly enough.

My Self Care Inventory

Feel free to steal any and certainly add your own.

Walking

I learned more about the East Side of Manhattan than I ever thought possible. The hospital is next to the East River, so I took several strolls to the water's edge, watching the boats drift by and letting the sound of the water work its magic on my muscles and psyche.

Doing Something for Others

The recreation area in the hospital had rolling carts of books that patients and visitors could take. As a book-a-holic, I noticed when the book inventory became depleted. I found a branch of the New York Public Library nearby that held an ongoing book sale. I purchased a boatload of books, hauled them back to the hospital and filled the sparsely laden book carts. It made me feel good to help out -- to give something back for the stellar care we received.

Do Something Fun for Yourself

At the time of Sally's treatment I was playing drums with a local band -- The Andy Browne Troupe. There was a scheduled gig that overlapped a stay in the hospital. I took a deep breath and left Sally in the care of her nurses and left for the day to play with the band.

Create Some Daily Downtime Rituals

Timing is everything. During Sally's treatment, all 13 seasons of MASH were available on Netflix. Every night in the hospital, I would grab something for dinner, sit somewhere quiet with my headphones plugged into my phone and watch my favorite MASH episodes. It was like visiting with old friends. Curiously, MASH disappeared from Netflix three weeks after Sally's final treatment. Something out there knew how to take care of me if I let it.

Scheduled Downtime

Being in the hospital was easy, there was an entire staff looking after Sally. It was being home where I went on-call twenty-four seven. That type of stress gets old quickly. I would call Sally's sister Katie and ask, "Can you come sit with Sally for two hours? I just need to get out for a bit." Katie never said "no." This was paramount especially in the early stages when Sally was still not communicating well and her coordination was suspect. Just getting in the car and driving around, grabbing a soda at WAWA, not being ON GUARD. It was enough to recharge my batteries for the next round of duty.

My self-care activities:

Notes:

Caregiver Tip #10

Get organized.

Knowledge has a calming effect. In the horrifying face of the unknown, the more you know, the better you will feel. All sorts of information, written and oral, is going to come at you trying to pierce the fog that has enveloped your life. Get a filing system in place that works for you. If nothing else this will be practice for the treatment phase and will make you feel a little more settled when it appears everything is spinning out of control.

"Take me home."

Sally's first tear-filled words after climbing in the car Sunday evening following the first six days at the hospital.

The daily blood-letting ritual was performed on schedule at two in the afternoon with the chemo level results due by four or so, the goal being to ensure Sally's chemo count was under 100. [1]

"What time is it?" Sally said, anxiously.

"A little after three. Give them a chance. Kristyn said between three-thirty and four is when the results usually come back."

"Think I can get dressed now?" Sally had reached her threshold for hospital stays. She wanted out. However, I knew she was trying to board the train before any ticket was issued, a sure-fire recipe for emotional disaster if her chemo count remained above 100. Even if the count was 101, that meant another 24 hours in-house until the next day's lab work was performed. Sally was convinced she was going, numbers be damned.

"Let's just wait until we are certain we are going. Let's wait to see what the number is," I said, which garnered a death-ray glare and a petulant pout.

It's easy to lose sight of the fact that Sloan delivered blood test results in two hours or less. Two hours, not three or four days. And on Sunday no less. In addition to the weekend staff we saw on the floor, I thought about all the people behind the scenes, lab techs, pathologists, etc., who also

---

[1] I could go into a lengthy monologue about what this number means and how it is derived but I'll spare you the med-speak. Just roll with it.

worked through the weekend. This fact, however, had little meaning to someone who had been poked, prodded and injected for six days straight.

By four-fifteen I thought Sally's head might explode. "What's the deal?" she kept asking, glaring at me.

"Patience."

"I am being patient. Tell them to hurry up already."

I just smiled and tried to model a calm demeanor. Internally, I was just as anxious, but I felt one of us had to remain reasonable, at least on the outside.

It was four eighteen when Kristyn appeared, staring at our anticipatory faces, and just blurted out, with her patented pixie grin, "39."

Sally set the Olympic Speed Packing record and crushed the world's best recorded time for changing from hospital gown into street clothes.

As part of the discharge process, Kristyn presented us with a grocery bag of medications and gave me the medication rundown for the next two weeks. "Sally takes this drug every six hours for 5 days. She takes this drug twice a day until the day before her next treatment. She takes this drug once a day but at a different time than the first drug. She takes this one only when the moon is full and the weekday has the letter "R" in the name...."

Honestly, I was only half paying attention as I thought, "Sure, sure, sure. Fine, fine. Can we go now?"

Well, almost – the patient had to be escorted to the front door by one of the nurses.

The plan: I get the car and bring it around front of the hospital. Remember to call when I get close as it's too cold to wait outside.

Nestled in behind the wheel for the first time in six days, I was shocked how wonderful it felt, mildly orgasmic. I love to drive and having not done so in six days left an unusual vacancy in my life, like not eating that last slab of tiramisu in the fridge because a visit to the doctor is a week away, and you need every advantage to keep from breaking his scale and incurring his wrath. Not that I have any experience with that.

Even on a Sunday, jostling through the taxis, hospital shuttles, EMS trucks, Halal food carts and other passenger pickups to grab someone in front of the hospital is like trying to ride a tricycle through full-throttle carnival bumper cars.

"Get back inside. It's cold," Sally said to Kristyn [2], giving her a hug and climbing in the car. Pulling back into the automotive chaos of East Side traffic, Sally's tears subsided into a sigh of immense relief.

Cross town traffic on 57th Street was always an experience. The trick is to think like a cab driver. Everywhere else in the US the motto is Drive Defensively, except New York City.[3] If you drive defensively in the Big Apple you'll get squashed. It's one of the few places where aggressive driving saves lives.

Weaving our way westward on 57th street, we approached 5th Avenue where, dangling 50-feet in the air was the UNICEF Crystal, a 28-foot, one and a half ton giant snowflake; a luminous beacon that declared its holiday intentions for blocks in every direction and to mark the location of every high-end jewelry store in the city. The upside to mid-town traffic was that we could spend time looking at something like this without whizzing by in a flash. I stared at the snowflake while waiting for the light to change, and the first ray of hope developed inside me. Unconsciously perhaps, the first inkling of seeing small things in a whole new light, and with a more significant appreciation, crept into my head.

---

2 Notice who tried to take care of whom while outside of the hospital room.
3 And Boston. Beantown drivers unnerve even me; I refuse to drive there without a full-body, flame retardant crash suit.

Home. We walked back in the door and after the dogs lost their minds at seeing us again, I reacquainted myself with the desk in the kitchen that had three weeks' worth of unpaid bills that needed to be sorted and one week's worth of unopened mail calling my name. On the wall above the desk was a small white board and above that a small blackboard, both featuring undecipherable drawings from the grandkids in an attempt to welcome us home. Upstairs I poked my head into my office and was disappointed to see the fairies had not straightened up the scattered work files and papers littering my small desk that also held two monitors, a scanner (upon which more file folders were stacked) and far too many desk tchotchkes; Play-Doh stars, Daffy Duck USB drive, Daffy Duck koosh ball, Daffy Duck mousepad (see the pattern here?), pens, trinkets etc., etc. In truth I had not given work much thought, life being more of a moment-by-moment prospect with all the new things we experienced.

With one treatment behind us, Sally's ability to speak, type, and think coherently did not come rushing back by magic, so the responsibility of meals, medications, dog care and on and on was now part of my life. Five minutes home and my head started gyrating as I suddenly realized what was in front of me. The lessons of my current job had thankfully drilled into me the idea of when faced with a mountain of stuff, prioritize and take one thing at a time.[4]

I immediately sat down with a pad and pen and sorted through the medication schedule for the following two weeks, creating a condensed andreadily understandable version of what had to be taken and when, just in case I got hit by a beer truck.[5]

---

4 All you multi-taskers can go pound sand.

5 Work also used the beer truck theory to describe a resource suddenly disappearing, allowing another person to easily assume the necessary tasks. Beer trucks being preferred over busses or trains; somehow it made the image of being squashed more palatable if alcohol was involved. Which it does.

I started getting glimpses of the amount of information coming our way and that I was responsible for maintaining it all. Little did I know at the time I was staring at the tip of the iceberg.

The discharge papers we received resembled the operating manual for any well-maintained nuclear power plant. I needed a translator. Nevertheless, I transcribed the medication directives into something even Gomer Pyle could comprehend:

	Dose	Start
Drug 1	1 pill three times a week	12/11
Drug 2	1 pill every six hours	12/12
Drug 3	1 injection every day if it rained	12/12
Drug 4	4mg for 4 days, then 3mg daily for two days, then "Pi r Squared" mg daily	12/14
Drug 5	17 grams dissolved in liquid daily if the Yankees hit a home run	12/14

The remaining five drugs were dosed out once a day.

As for the one drug that had to be taken every six hours, I realized it didn't matter how that was timed, at some point I was going to have to drag my ass out of a warm bed and onto a cold floor to make sure we didn't miss feeding time.

Next priority item: shopping list.

Up until this point, I'd been stuffing all the paperwork we'd been receiving into one of those scholastic folders with pockets good for about fifteen sheets of paper. I carted around not only prescription documents, but also all the lab reports and MRI discs from every scan, test and inquisition Sally had endured. It was getting tougher to keep track of everything, so the first item on the list was an expandable fan folder of some consequence and a

CD/DVD travel case. Well, maybe second thing on the shopping list as we had been gone for six days and needed to hit the grocery store. Sally's sister Katie had made some soup and some dinner for our return home, but the cupboards were a bit bare.

But Scarlett, tomorrow is another day. We showered, scraping off six days of hospital, and headed for bed.

Think of the best sex you have ever had or quenching a deep thirst on a hot day with the coldest, best tasting drink imaginable. After six days in a sleeper chair, lying in bed felt like all of that and more. Sally and I looked at each other, smiling, but didn't say a word; it was one of those moments that we wished could last forever. I made a vow to my pillow to never take it for granted again. With Sydney and Slater intertwined around our legs, sleep wrapped us up and took us away, at least until the next medication alarm sounded.

According to research statistics, the average caregiver can expect to spend 13 days a month on tasks such as shopping, food preparation, housekeeping, laundry, transportation, and giving medication. So, roughly 78 hours a week. Well let's break that down...

Activity	Hours Required	Hours Remaining
Available hours in a week		168
Sleep	56	112
Work	40 (stop laughing)	72
Caregiving	78	**Oh shit....**
The rest of your life	???	**What the...**

Okay. So much for statistics.

After medications were downed and breakfast consumed[6] the next eight hours were spent in typical Monday fashion: reading emails and listening to conference calls without accomplishing anything substantial.

Sally slept most of the day feeling okay but wiped out. I was checking the drug schedule in between-conference calls, letting my paranoia about missing something take control.

I asked Katie to stop by after she got off work and babysit, so to speak, while Sally slept so I could venture to the grocery store. We live in an area where 55-plus retirement homes flourish, so most of the narrow aisles at the local Shop-Rite inevitably resemble the motorized scooter version of a monster truck rally.

While dashing from aisle to aisle -- where do they hide the damn peanut butter anyway? -- I quickly learned that one essential piece of clothing needed to blast through the grocery store are reverse shin guards. The bumpers on those scooters are hell on my heels and Hell's Grannies have no qualms about running your ass over if they think you are spending entirely too much time choosing a brand of canned tuna. I started losing track of what I had in my shopping cart. Frozen veggies, cereal, dog food, pretzels, dog food, soup, Pampers…how the hell did those get in there?? I was so involved in taking cart inventory that as I exited the snacks aisle I had to slam on the brakes to avoid being t-boned by a maroon and black scooter decorated with a skull and crossbones decal and driven by a tiny, skeletal woman with a black bandanna wrapped around her head who flipped me off and gave out a high pitched cackle at the look of terror in my face.[7]

I narrowly escaped into the health aids aisle in search of two thing I knew we needed:

---

6 Can't call the food service people for breakfast though. Damn. Guess there's an upside to everything.

7 Well…that's what I thought I saw…

Hand Sanitizer[8]

I grabbed a couple Big Gulp-sized bottles and then a couple pocket-sized ones thinking I could refill from the big ones. That thought made me feel smart. It's the little victories that matter. Germs are the enemy of patients with compromised immune systems. The hospital had a hand sanitizer dispenser about every six feet on the wall of every corridor. Home would require more effort.

Sanitizing wipes

These suckers may kill germs but left my hands smelling like a heavily chlorinated swimming pool. And from the Little Known Facts file, the germ killing action of sanitizing wipes does not come from the wipe itself, it comes from the post-application drying action. Once you wipe down a surface, let it dry on its own. If you wipe up with a dry towel immediately after using the sanitary wipe, the germ-killing benefits are negated. It may look like a trail of slime remains behind, but resist the urge to clean it up. Feel free to use this new knowledge to impress your friends and relatives.

I cautiously merged into the bumper-to-bumper traffic queued up in the checkout line. Six million people and five registers were open. While waiting and thinking of all the other tasks I could be accomplishing, I overheard the following from a passing father whose teenage daughter was pushing the shopping cart:

Daughter: "Oh cool! You got marshmallows!"
Father - with pained expression: "Those are not marshmallows, they're cotton balls."

---

8 Once again, this is all pre-COVID when these items were on hardly anyone else's radar.

I laughed out loud, which garnered a lot of evil looks. I didn't care. A little humor would get me through even grocery shopping insanity.

I got home, unpacked, took the dogs for a walk while Katie was still there. Cooked dinner, fed the hounds, made sure the meds were on schedule, threw in a load of laundry, and cleaned up the dinner dishes. Some roller skates would really have helped.

It was about nine at night when I finally sat down and…did nothing. Exhaustion took over. In my growing stupor, it dawned on me that it's no wonder women with kids don't want to have sex. They're too friggin' tired. Hubby comes home from "a hard day at the office" of megalomaniacal bosses, whining co-workers, phone calls and attending some unknown co-worker's birthday where free cake can be snatched, and can't understand why Mom doesn't want to get funky after the kids are asleep.

Shopping list:

Creative Organizational Ideas:

Notes:

Caregiver Tip # 11

Holidays will be different. Plan ahead.

Being in the hospital is bad enough; throw a holiday - any holiday - in the mix and the emotional temperature of the experience gets an additional kick in the ass. Here is where additional forethought comes into play. Get creative - not overblown (unless that's your style) just creative.

ASK FOR HELP
(sound familiar yet?)

We spent four holidays in-patient: Valentine's Day, Independence Day, Thanksgiving and Christmas.

Round two of chemotherapy started on December 10th. From the hospital window, I looked out at the cold December day, layers of grey clouds hung like wet cotton over the East River; whether they produced rain, sleet or snow was still up for grabs. As the treatment routine took over, I spent more time wandering the hospital corridors and streets of the city, trying to figure out how I was going to emotionally and physically handle the upcoming Christmas holiday.

I had already figured out on the calendar that our bi-weekly chemo routine was laid out to ensure the third round of treatment would start with an out-patient visit to the Basking Ridge infusion center on December 23rd, then traveling to New York on Christmas Eve Day and spending Christmas Day pumped full of chemo in an advanced state of depression. How was I going to create a Christmas where we were surrounded by family and friends when Sally required limited exposure to others due to her increasingly compromised immune system? Every year we traveled to either Katie's or Chris's house on Christmas Eve where Santa (me) read "The Night Before Christmas" to the younger kids. Then there was a trip to my sister's house to celebrate with my side of the family. And, of course, Christmas Day with our own kids and grandkids. And those are just the physical traditions.

Christmas shopping was going to fall on me as well this year; Sally's exposure to sniffling and sneezing holiday shoppers had to be minimized, if not forbidden. Sally and I have an annual tradition where a Christmas budget is determined, figuring in brothers, sisters, kids, grandkids, nephews, nieces, boyfriends, girlfriends and any passersby who needs a place to hang for the holidays. We stick to this budget until approximately December 15th when one of us will cross the line with "Fuck it, it's Christmas" and proceed to max out our credit cards with gift buying. When our kids were growing up, I was usually the first to cross the pre-determined budget line much to Sally's consternation, she being the keeper of the checkbook. Now, with the grandkids, Grandma breaks the "Fuck it, it's Christmas" budget sometime around August seventh, long before an actual number is even established. When it comes to her grandkids, just get out of the way. So, the prospect of not being able to partake in the traditional activities of Christmas shopping, not having the energy to decorate, and spending the second consecutive family holiday in the hospital weighed heavily on Sally. What could I do to keep her spirits up?

As I aimlessly wandered the hospital corridors, head spinning and allowing the current situation to gain exponential weight on every muscle of my neck and shoulders, I suddenly realized I was standing in the middle of Santa's Workshop.

Deep in the bowels of the hospital's main building, the maintenance team dwelled; the windowless, dark hallways ceilinged with pipes, wires, and ductwork. In December, however, the hallways transformed into hundreds of twinkling lights, life-sized cutouts of snowmen, Snoopy, Rudolph, and Christmas elves. A working train platform was constructed in one corner by the service elevator. My thoughts flipped to the kids who were stuck in the hospital fighting the good fight instead of being home with friends and family getting psyched for Santa's arrival. Hopefully, the ambulatory kids were able to come down and visit the decorations, to bring some Christmas spirit into their lives. My body shook with chills. There is a special courage exhibited by kids with cancer and their parents. It's a bravery that far eclipses what my fertile mind can imagine, not to mention the complete heartbreak of seeing bald children wheeled through the corridors hooked up to IV drips and donning face masks.

Just then my phone rang; Beth's number showed on the call screen.

"Hey, what's up?" I said, happy to have my thoughts interrupted.

"I have a question for you. I was talking with Aunt Kate, and we want to decorate your house. You know, put up lights and stuff so Mom has it all there when she comes home. What do you think?"

It never dawned on me to ask for help ...

(DDDUUUUUUHHHHHHH!)

Even though decorating was traditionally something Sally and I did together, I did the outside lights, she took care of inside the house, I had come to the conclusion that decorating was just not going to happen this year. I couldn't see how it was going to get done in light of everything else going on. And if we were going to spend Christmas Day in the hospital, why bother?

A surge of energy coursed through me. "Absolutely," I said, eyes welling up. "That would be awesome."

Beth said, "Don't tell Mom."

"That'll be perfect. She'll see them as we drive up to the house."

Surrounded by Santa's Workshop in the basement of Sloan Kettering, I felt some of the weight disappear, my muscles loosened a bit. A little Christmas spirit unexpectedly wormed its way in.

The neon lit streets of the East Side provided another unexpected surprise: the smell of Christmas trees. Live tree concessions dot the corners every couple blocks and the evergreen smell was pungent, mixing with the odor of roasted chestnuts from street vendors. I expected to find Nat King Cole standing on a corner crooning The Christmas Song. The evergreen scent reminded me of Christmas tree shopping as a kid, walking through the annual YMCA Christmas tree sale set up on the field across from the Elm Street school. As crazy as my house was growing up, the days between Thanksgiving and Christmas were always fun and exciting; the memories I have of that time soothed me further as I bustled through the evening crowds of First Avenue.

Christmas in Manhattan. Sure it's crowded, cold and crazy, but it is also spectacularly decorated. It also drives home the need to be grateful. I stopped at the bank for some cash and was greeted by a homeless man keeping warm by napping in the bank/ATM lobby. As if I hadn't been handed enough blessings recently.

Sally cleared the chemo for round two quickly, so we were able to return home on Saturday the 13th. The customary checkout time was five-ish in the afternoon, so by the time we got our bag of goodies from the nurses, and I battled traffic to pick her up on York Ave in front of the hospital, the sky was dark and the Christmas lights of Manhattan had ignited.

As we passed under the UNICEF snowflake on Fifty-Seventh and Fifth, we were reminded that we made it through another treatment; I was suddenly overcome with a deep-rooted feeling that everything was going to be okay.

Once through the tunnel and into New Jersey there was a palpable sigh of relief, not unlike rafting through white water and emerging on a glassine stream. The next level of relaxation started to kick in.

Tooling down the turnpike, Sally talked about all the things she wanted to get done, now that there were less than two weeks before Christmas. Her action list included all the shopping and decorating she would do under normal circumstances.

"It's going to be different this year," I said as gently as possible. "You can't be running around in the stores, and you won't have the energy to get all you want done. I can do some and Beth can do some. You're going to have to lean on us this year."

Glassy-eyed, she said "I know. But I can go out sometimes, can't I?"

"We can go to a couple places as long as it's off hours so the crowds will be minimal. But you can't drive yet, and the last thing we need is for you to catch something."

Caretakers often have to be the voice of reality, even if it's repeating sucky news the patients do not want to hear, especially patients who go fiveyears-old during the holidays.

As we pulled off Route 130 onto Main Street Cranbury, Sally said, "What's so funny?"

"Huh?"

"You have a big shit-eating grin on your face."

I had to think of something quick. My anticipation of Sally seeing our house decorated broke through, and I didn't want to spoil the surprise.

"Just glad to be home. You know, getting off the highway and back into town. Hey, look at the houses all lit up."

In my favor was Sally's innate characteristic to trust just about everything I say. There are many who would not let me get away with a lame redirect like that.

Remember The Andy Griffith Show? That's where we lived. Even the locals refer to it as Mayberry.

As with most New Jersey towns, about 50 percent of the houses, a combination of new construction on the outskirts surrounding historically preserved Revolutionary War era homes, were decorated for St. Nick in some fashion. We slowed down as we passed that house that has embraced the glitzy, dance club trend Christmas extravaganza with flashing LED lights covering the roof, the lawn, a hand-built, two-story light-wall, and a flagpole draped in lights to resemble a Chirstmas tree. The schedule for the pull-all-the-stops-out gonzo presentation is posted in front of the house with No Parking signs posted every hundred feet for a quarter mile in each direction to make sure drive-by gawkers don't cause fender-benders or run over Ritalin-stoked kids tweaked into a frenzy by the epileptic lights.

"That's a project I wouldn't want to tackle. I have enough trouble getting the grass cut on a regular basis."

"It's a bit much," Sally said as we continued to gawk.

Two houses away from the blazing showplace we passed a house decorated with life size plywood cutouts of Snoopy's doghouse and figures of Charlie Brown, Linus and Woodstock, the diorama lit by a single spotlight and fronted with a sign reading, "A Christmas Un-Spectacular." "Nothing like Christmas to bring out neighborhood ideological battles," I said.

"Too funny."

We turned the corner to enter our street; I kept a peripheral eye on Sally. I spotted the lights, but it took a minute for what she saw to register, and then for her to start crying.

"Oh, my God," she sobbed.

The front of the house was ablaze with our favorite Christmas decoration scheme, a combination of white and colored strings wrapped around the columns of the front porch and outlining the front door. In each window the yellowish glow of electric candles radiates, the same candles we had been using since before the kids were born. We pulled in the driveway and sat, Sally just letting it wash over her.

"What…" was all she could say.

I revealed the plot cooked up by Katie, Jimmy, Beth and Stephen. "They know how much Christmas means to you and didn't want you to miss it."

Suitcases in tow, we headed through the side door to the welcoming committee of two crazy dogs, overjoyed with our return. Wading through dog slobber, we entered the den. This time even I was surprised and moved. Sally stopped and started crying again when she saw the fresh-cut Christmas tree standing in the corner, complete with lights. I expected the house lights, but they really went above and beyond.

I found a note our Christmas elves had left in the kitchen.

"They purposely left the ornaments off, knowing how much you wanted to decorate it with the grandkids," I said summarizing what I read.

Sally was a speechless wreck. The indoor fichus tree was also decorated with lights, another tradition, and a handful of other decorations had been unpacked and scattered throughout the house. Those we love can do amazing things if we let them.

The biggest Christmas gift we received came a few days later.

Sally sat in the kitchen sifting through the mail, the omnipresent mug of tea in front of her. She held a greeting card of some sort and was reading it with a glassy-eyed stare.

"Christmas cards already?" I felt a small twinge of guilt. Christmas cards. When was I going to have time for that?

"No," she said. "It's a card from Tom and Jane. There's a quote, 'Scared is what you're feeling. Brave is what you are doing.'" She read Jane's note. "Sally, you and Jim are showing us a courage we can only imagine. We love you and are sending our prayers to you every day." Aside from the wonderful card, I felt a spark of hope; I could see inklings of comprehension starting to come back for Sally. I wasn't sure if it was the chemo or the steroids, but I was happy to see her ability to read something and discern its meaning.

Even so, I was still in charge of communicating with all the doctors and maintaining the schedule of treatments and checkups.

I sat at the kitchen table next to Sally and said, "I just got off the phone with Dr. G's office."

Sally wears her emotions on her face; I could see she was bracing herself for something she didn't want to hear. "Yeah?"

"They said the start of next round of treatment can be pushed from the 23rd to the 26th. Merry Christmas!"

This produced tears but a huge smile. "We're going to be able to spend Christmas at home with the family?" she asked.

"To the extent we can, yes."

I could not have asked for anything better in order to keep Sally's spirits up.

What I didn't expect was that friends from the distant past would also bestow a few heartfelt gifts. Our friends from high school, rekindled through social media and the reunion, applied their talents to keep Sally going.

"Something for you in the mail," I said to Sally, handing her a small, rectangular box.

"What is it?" She asked.

"No idea. I don't recognize the return address either, but it's North Jersey."

Opening the package Sally pulled out a large wooden ornament in the shape of an old-fashioned key about a foot long and painted blue, with a heart for a handle. Two tiny snowmen and various stars and snowflakes were handprinted across the surface; on the back it was signed "RVS '74".

As an independent senior year project, one of our high school classmates, Rosie V. put together a talent show (*Hey Kids let's put on a show!!!*). For the finale, all the performers came out on stage to sing, "Prepare Ye The Way of The Lord" from Godspell, which was big at the time. Rosie asked me to play drums for the finale and being the stage-ham I was at the time, I readily accepted. Now, after 40 years of no contact, Rosie had taken the time to hand-make something to cheer Sally up through her journey. Out of nowhere. We hung it next to our backdoor, the one we use most often, to make us smile every day.

A couple days later, another box arrived, this one a bit larger and from the address I knew it was from our friends Rich and Jill. I had known Rich since ninth grade, we went to college together and he was the best man at our wedding.

"Look at all this stuff," Sally said. "You guys…". Sally said "you guys" whenever she was blown away by something, even if the givers were nowhere near. From the box Sally extracted a winter hat and a long snake.

"What the hell is that?" I asked.

"It's a neck warmer. You put it in the microwave then wrap it around your neck to keep warm," she said, modeling the accoutrement for me.

The next day, "Package for you, Lady!" I said, returning from the mailbox. "You need your own post office branch. This is crazy."

"Oh wow," Sally said, rummaging through a box full of different dry skin lotions and potions. "Who is this from," she said pulling out a note from the box and reading, "'From previous experience I know these are perfect to help along your journey. Enjoy. Dina.'

"Who's Dina?"

Dina J. was a woman with whom I worked who apparently had previous experience with this kind of odyssey and wanted to tangibly show her support. The amazing part is that Dina had never met Sally. The gesture moved me as much as Sally.

There was one more box yet to arrive, but this one I knew about.

On Christmas Eve, a bundle of love arrived. Sally stood in the kitchen trying to untie the heavy twine keeping the package together, thankfully she avoided impaling her palm with a steak knife and opted to use scissors, not that she was any safer wielding those. She folded back the layers of tissue paper.

"Oh my God. Oh my God. Cooper, look… It's beautiful."

One of our more bohemian high school friends was Nancy K (now W), a zoftig Earth Mother with an unmistakable laugh, a gentle soul and a massive capacity for love. She too was a drama geek. She too was someone we lost touch with for 40 years and discovered she married another classmate and drama-tech guy Jeff W. There was something about Nancy that we always connected with – although I would venture to say Nancy is one of those people who can instantly connect with anyone who is decent and has a big heart. One of her specialties is sewing gorgeous patchwork quilts by hand, a square at a time, customizing each for her lucky recipients. She had decided to make one for Sally.

I promised Nancy I would video the unveiling. Sally unfolded the beautiful hand-made blanket saying, "How can she do this?" Looking at the camera, she said "Thank you, Nancy."

I pointed out, "There's a heart on the back that has something written on it." Flipping it all around Sally found the white sewn-on heart that read, "You are loved. By Nancy W. 12-14"

Sally put it on our bed straight away, and there it stayed. The heart and soul that went into this gift was a viable force, helping Sally to heal every time she got in bed.

That night, Sally's entire family gathered at her sister Kate's house to celebrate. It was the first time in quite awhile that all Sally's nieces and nephews, including our own kids, were gathered together in one place. I could not have asked for a better tonic.

Christmas Day was quiet, which was different for us, but somehow felt right. Our kids were suddenly "older" and had girlfriend/boyfriend families to take into account. They were with us only part of the day, so there was an unusual amount of quiet in the house. I still felt incredibly lucky. From a caregiver perspective, I sat back and let things happen; friends and family rose to the occasion and helped bring Sally all the Christmas spirit they could muster. I realized all I needed to do was give up some control and get the hell out of the way.

To-do list for any upcoming holiday:

_____
_____
_____
_____
_____
_____
_____
_____
_____
_____
_____
_____

People that can help for the upcoming holiday:

_____
_____
_____
_____
_____
_____
_____
_____

Notes:

Caregiver Tip #12

Find distractions to minimize the constant medical focus - for the patient and yourself

The 24/7 focus on all things cancer is at best wearing and at most mentally debilitating. Distractions are a necessary part of keeping sane for both the caregiver and the patient. Finding them requires stepping out of your brain and re-connecting to the world around you. Easier said than done with the constant focus on all things cancer.

Sally's ennui grew with each treatment, bolstered by staring at linoleum floors and cramped quarters, listening to the incessant IV monitor beeping, and staring at repetitive television drudgery. In one sense we were grateful that the treatments were uneventful. In another sense time in the hospital was desperately dull and boring. Anything that caught my eye in my travels through the halls or in the streets was fodder for distracting Sally and me away from the stress and boredom of treatment. For example:

The Twilight Zone Elevator

"What's the matter?" Sally asked as I sat in the sleeper chair, a look of consternation on my face.

"I'm okay. Just had a bizarre elevator experience. I got on the first floor and pushed seven, but the button for the second floor lit up."

"Did it stop on two?" she asked.

"Yeah. I pushed seven again after the doors closed and the three button came on. Same thing happened, it stopped on three."

At this point Kristyn came in to take Sally's vitals.

"When the same thing happened on four, I jumped out and walked the rest of the way. I was afraid it was going to break loose at any second and free fall, crashing into splinters at the bottom of the shaft, or possibly shift into fourth gear and go rocketing through the top of the shaft a la Willy Wonka."

"That's weird," Sally said

Kristyn chimed in, "The elevator?" I nodded. "That's just the Sabbath elevator."

"More like the Black Sabbath elevator," I said

"Orthodox Judaism prohibits the touching of certain items during the Sabbath. Every Friday the Sabbath elevator stops at every floor in both directions continually so the floor buttons don't need to be touched."

"Some sort of sign for us clueless goyim would be nice," I said.

It's a twister! It's a twister!

We were between chemo rounds six and seven, in the heart of February's grey depression on life. Treatments were tougher, as nausea appeared, and Sally exhibited zero appetite outside of ice cream and coffee cake. In between hospital stays, cabin fever was a constant visitor as trips outside were seriously curtailed with the flu season in full swing and Sally's immune system getting clobbered on a bi-weekly basis.

In addition, my nursing duties took a more active role. I was in the kitchen washing and sanitizing my hands. "It's time," I said.

Sally groaned and grudgingly exposed her stomach in preparation for the injection I had to administer to keep at least a nominal level of white cells ready for action.

As much as I tried to be gentle, the pain level of my injections ranged from not-too-bad to holy-shit-that-hurt.

"All set?" I said.

"Just do it."

I sanitized a patch of skin, pinched a small patch and plunged the needle into her. I saw in Sally's face that this was not one of my better efforts and she was at the point of reaching her limit with…everything. The medicines, the grey weather, feeling crappy, cooped up in the house; it was all coming to a head.

"Come on. Get your coat," I said.

Sally looked at me quizzically. "Where are we going? It's two in the afternoon."

I herded her into the car and took off. Just getting outside revitalized her spirits to a small degree. "Let's go," I said after we parked at the local movie octo-plex.

"The movies? What are we seeing?"

"You'll see."

We sat in the theater, watched a small clip featuring the late Robert Osborne, the Lion roared and the wind whipped into a frenzy as the munchkin chorus introduced the opening strains to The Wizard of Oz.

"Oh, cool!" Sally said, a big grin on her face.

Turner Classic Movies was sponsoring a theatrical release of one of Sally's favorites. I opted for a weekday afternoon showing anticipating a small crowd, or at least a smaller one. We sat in the nearly deserted theater watching Dorothy and Toto cavort on the big screen. It made for a welcome break for both of us.

Forward, Into the Past!

A double-sided, standard issue, schoolroom clock with a red, sweeping second hand protruded from the wall of each hospital corridor. One day, more out of habit than timekeeping, I glanced up at the timepiece and just as quickly kept walking, until the time delay between my eye and my brain stopped me in my tracks. After stepping backwards several steps, further examination confirmed that not only was the time displayed incorrectly, but also that the second hand was running…backwards. I stood and stared at it for the better part of 30 seconds, making sure I wasn't hallucinating. I stepped ahead to look at the other side of the clock. That side functioned correctly.

One of the cleaning people exited a room across the hall, and gave me a wayward glance, certainly wondering what this fool was up to, just standing in the middle of the hallway staring at the clock.

"Take a look at this," I said motioning her to my side. Hesitantly she joined me, staring up at the timepiece. After a full 15 seconds of silence, I said, "Why is it running backwards?"

She cast a suspicious glance my way. "I don't know," she said and walked away, shaking her head and chuckling. "Don't be messing with me. I can't take it."

I stood there for a few minutes more, grabbing nurses and anyone else who would hear me out, about the reverse timepiece. Perhaps it had some practical medical purpose of which I was not yet acquainted. No one, however, had a rational explanation. The general reaction was a smirk and a shake of the head, as if to say, "Yeah. No surprise there."

Upon entering Sally's room I said, "You've got to come see this."

We were in the midst of treatment six and aside from feeling nauseous, Sally was getting fed up with sitting around in bed doing nothing. She looked at me as if I had asked her to run the New York City marathon. Eventually she disentangled her IV tubes, got out of bed, rolling IV stand and all, and followed me to the clock.

"Oh, that's weird," she said with a smirk, which I took as a small victory.

Aerial Acrobatics

"You're 90 to 95 percent clear," Dr. G. told us after the originally scheduled eight chemo treatments. "I want to do two more rounds to see if we can knock it all out."

Good news, bad news. Even though we were missing all of our nurse and nurse practitioner buddies at the hospital, returning for additional treatments was not the circumstances upon which we wanted to return. Sally was flat-out bummed at the prospect of more chemo.

Our seventh-floor suite for treatment number nine afforded us a northern view of York Avenue, which also looked down on the empty lot across 68th Street that was surrounded with construction fences and fancy artist renderings of the swanky new hospital facility to be built there.

"Hey, check this out," I said, staring out of the window.

We watched lego-sized construction workers build a three-story crane on York Avenue, and then use the three-story crane to hoist tangles of white steel that fit together to form a tower, not unlike Lego blocks.

"What is that?" Sally asked fascinated with the construction ballet.

"I don't know. Maybe a frame for a construction elevator?"

As we watched over the course of the afternoon, the white steel evolved into a larger crane's column structure, that was topped with the operator's box, and then the lengthy crane arm.

However, the curtain rose the following day on the real show.

We watched the yellow, hard-hatted construction crew creep over the towering skeleton, like spiders knitting a massive web, six stories in the air, to attach the operating cables stretching all the way to the end of the crane arm.

"Holy crap," I said, in awe. By this time, I had positioned the visitor chairs to face the window providing a more comfortable gawking space. "You could not pay me enough to do that."

Dressed in a hospital gown and robe, and IV tubes tethering her to a rolling stand replete with bags of cancer killers and multiple IV monitors, Sally watched through the window, fascinated by the dangerous choreography on steel across the street. It certainly beat staring at the TV all day.

Fun distractions:

Notes:

Caregiver Tip # 13

Celebrate everything...
no matter how small.

"Look for small victories and build on that. Each small victory, even if it is just getting up five minutes earlier, gives you confidence. You realize that these little victories make you feel great, and you keep going. You realize that being paralyzed by fear of failure is worse than failure."
- Arnold Schwarzenegger

Dr. G. said, "Count backwards from one hundred. By sevens."
Sevens? Seriously?

I held my breath waiting for Sally to give this a shot. We were in the hospital for the pre-chemo checkup prior to round six. Chemo's routine had produced a sense of security for me. Unlike pre-diagnosis where not knowing pushed me as close to living in a padded room as I ever care to be, there was a comfort in not knowing during the chemo treatments, that the next check inside Sally's head was weeks away and not something I needed to think about. Call it a resurgence in denial, but until the eighth treatment was complete and the first MRI would be taken to see what impact all the drugs Sally was ingesting had made, I felt at ease letting the medical community do its thing.

Prior to the sixth treatment, however, a status of Sally's symptoms would be gauged for the first time since treatment began. By this time, steroids had been completely removed from Sally's daily medication intake. Dr. G. had been weaning her off them since the second treatment and by the sixth treatment, Sally had been steroid-free for three weeks.

The pre-check-up tension, which is part and parcel of the process, was ratcheted up for this one.

We sat waiting, and sweating, in the examination room until Dr. G. appeared.

"I want you to remember three things," he said. "Ready? Thirty-five, red rooster, Miami." He asked Sally to repeat them back, which she did. A good start.

"Okay. Spell "world" backwards."

Sally concentrated for a minute. She had never been able to get completely through this. "D..L...", she said, hesitating again. I was holding my breath. "R..O..W."

"Excellent," Dr. G. said, visibly impressed. I was smiling from ear to ear – the first time she completed that unaided.

"Is that right?" Sally said, also somewhat surprised.

"You got it," Dr. G. said. I thought Sally was going to jump up and dance. "Now, how many nickels in $1.35." Oh this was a new one. I flashed back to Sally trying to teach Beth the value of money by showing her a quarter, a nickel, and three pennies, telling her it was thirty-eight cents. No kidding – we have it captured on video.

Sally thought for awhile. I could see the wheels spinning in her head. Even I had to do some quick head-math to figure it out.

Dr. G. said, "How many nickels in a dollar? How many nickels in thirty-five cents?"

"Twenty-seven!" Sally blurted out.

"Exactly." Now I was really impressed.

"One more, count backwards from one-hundred. By sevens."

Holy crap!

"Okay. One hundred. Ninety-three." A slight pause. "Eighty-six."

Dr. G. nodded. "Uh-huh. Keep going."

"Seventy-nine. Seventy-two." Another pregnant pause. I was silently doing the same math but not coming up with the answers all that much faster than Sally. "Umm. Sixty…five?"

Dr. G. nodded again.

"Fifty.eight," she said with some confidence this time.

"Yeah, that's good enough," Dr. G. said. "Good work."

After putting Sally though the usual motion tests of walking a straight line, heel-to-toe, comparing right and left leg pressure and peripheral vision, he said, "Okay. What are the three things I asked you to remember?"

She looked kind of blank for a couple seconds, as if trying to recall some distant memory.

"Red rooster."

"Uh-huh."

A pause. "Thirty-five."

A longer pause. Dr. G. said, "A place."

"Miami!" she said. That was the first time she remembered all three.

Dr. G. was happy with her progress. We had smiles a mile wide.

Afterward, we sat inside the car in the hospital parking lot and made immediate phone calls to Kate, Stephen and Beth. This was big stuff – Sally's brain was starting to function without steroids, and better than it had in over a year.

This called for an immediate celebratory lunch. Our usual post-visit stop was the Chimney Rock Inn. I ordered a beer. When the waitress asked Sally what she wanted,

"A really big Diet Coke." Her standard response.

After being served, I held my beer up in toast. "Congratulations. This is big stuff, and you are killing it." We clinked glasses.

"I don't feel like I'm doing anything." This, too, was a common Sally comment.

"More than you know. If nothing else, you are showing the rest of us how this is done. That's huge." She looked at me suspiciously, as if I had just casually mentioned that the sky was a lovely shade of green.

Sometimes though, the need for celebration is not as clear-cut, especially to the patient, and as the caregiver, I had to look for ways to make sure milestones were not ignored, regardless of the current diagnosis.

Treatment seven was the first major checkpoint; that's when Dr. G. would peek under the hood with the first MRI since the chemo dance began. In the midst of number seven, I started feeling anxious; some of the initial "not-knowing" anxiety started weighing on me. Before number seven, I didn't have to worry about a progress report. It was simply a matter of trusting that the doctors knew what they were doing. Now we stared in the face of "is all of this really working?" I was somewhat buoyed by Sally's progress symptom-wise, functioning steroid-free for several weeks without any relapses in speech or motor issues.

We silently sat in the examination room engulfed in skin-crawling tension as we waited for Dr. G.'s pronouncement. If you think time moved slowly when you were in third grade….

"So," Dr. G. said upon entering. "The cancer is about 85 - 90 % gone, which is great."

I didn't feel like it was great. I was hoping for the 100% everyone said was going to happen. Judging by her expression, Sally was feeling a bit confused as well. "Soooooo….." I said, in hopes of hearing a good next step.

"I want to do two more rounds of chemo."

Sally's disappointment was palpable. "Really?" she said, discouraged.

Dr. G. explained. "There's just a little bit left, and I want to kick it out of there. We'll do an MRI after each one to check on progress."

It wasn't what we had hoped for, but it was light years from where we started. We gathered ourselves up, called everyone in the family putting on a positive spin, that the cancer was almost all gone and how great was that?

Once we returned home, I made another phone call to our daughter Beth. "It's time," I said. "Come over tonight."

Later that evening, Sally was still coming to terms with the extra chemo treatments; she had her heart and mind thoroughly set on "seven," so the extra visits were laying heavily on her soul.

Suddenly, the side door burst open and our two grandkids exploded into the room, jumping on the sofa into Sally's lap.

"Mom-Mom! Mom-Mom!!" This was the first time she had seen them in about three months. It was the best thing I could think of to celebrate her remarkable progress and lift her spirits at the same time.

Things to be celebrated:

_____
_____
_____
_____
_____
_____
_____
_____
_____
_____

Ways to celebrate:

_____
_____
_____
_____
_____
_____

Notes:

Caregiver Tip #14

> Doctors are the mechanics.
> Nurses are the healers.
> Treat them as such.

Nurses are crazy. No rational thinking human being should willingly do what these people do on a daily basis. It must be a genetic flaw. Whatever it is, a world populated with this type of insanity would be utopia.

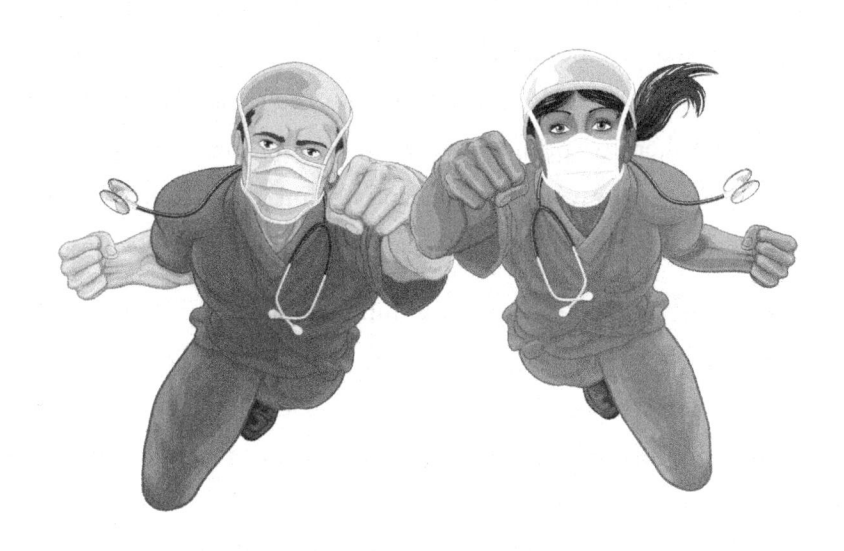

Things You Have to Love to Be a Nurse

1) Insomnia - especially if you have any intention of leading the semblance of a normal social existence. Think back to any all-nighters you have pulled, triple it, and then follow it by three days of complete inertia.

2) Communal living - Wage-slave, corporate types thrive on cube space, the bigger the better, the more removed the better (anyone with a cube facing a well-travelled hallway or, horrors, the bosses office has "short-timer" written all over it). It's a matter of power and status, one's cube space. Nurses? Forget about it. They live out their days in the bullpen, a vast space of constant traffic, unrelenting noise and mass hysteria. That's their sanctuary. Not even locking themselves in the john will provide any privacy because there are probably only two or three bathrooms on the floor, and some idiot is always walking by and jiggling the handle, even if the red "occupied" flag is showing. And speaking of which...

3) Pee and poop - Nurses are mind-numbingly obsessed with urine and excrement, much like Moses was obsessed with radical shortcuts. The obsession is not steeped in narcissism; they are enthralled by EVERYONE's pee and poop: how much, the last evacuation event, consistency. Any discussion concerning laxatives and stool softeners creates a glazed look in a nurse's eye equal to walking up to a cat and dangling a PCP laced catnip mouse in its face.

4) Whining - Nurses become semi-orgasmic at the sound of other people's critical issues, such as,

- My room is too hot
- My room is too cold
- My roommate is an asshole
- The food sucks
- No-one made my bed today
- My son the doctor says you're doing this wrong

If it weren't for the patients, the nurses would be having a really great time. We did our best to be "good patients," for their sanity and ours. Sometimes, though, shit happens. For example, our post-fourth round treatment escape became legend within the nurse community. It wasn't a premeditated AWOL, we just cracked under the pressure, having been saddled with demanding roommates, including a husband with whom I played sleeper chair bumper cars throughout the night. Sally and I didn't sleep much during this particular 72-hour visit, consequently, we looked and felt like extras on the set of The Walking Dead. Or models from the Sephora store. Same thing.

This was the first time Sandra had been assigned as Sally's nurse. She was a red-headed force of nature from Long Island.[1]

"You guys are good to go," Sandra said on the afternoon of day three, letting us know Sally's chemo numbers were low enough that we could flee. So we did just that; changed, packed up and left. We made our way down to the first floor corridor, in a fog, headed for the parking garage.

(First ignored hint – the nurses always escort patients to the pick-up point on York Ave.).

---

1 Think The Sopranos meets Two Broke Girls

As we made our way, we ran into Fariel who almost immediately said, "You still have your pic line?"

We both looked at Sally's arm, and sure as shit her pic line still dangled from the back of her hand.

(Second ignored hint – how the hell did that happen?)

Fariel reached into her pockets for some sterile wipes and a band aid[2] and fixed Sally up.

Five o'clock on Friday evening leaving the city. We were going nowhere fast, having to traverse the entire island on 57th, Street and then head for the Lincoln Tunnel. By the time we hit the Jersey Turnpike, which included a dazed, errant detour turning onto Tenth Avenue the wrong way into rush hour traffic, we were burnt to a crisp.

Then my phone rang. Having previously shelled out $150 for a "using cell while driving" summons, I was not in the habit of answering behind the wheel, but the phone number had a 212 area code. The only 212 calls I received were from Sloan.

"Hello?" I said.

"Mr. Cooper? This is Sandra. Where are you?"

I let her know where we were.

"But I didn't discharge you! We've been looking all over for you. I have all your prescriptions. You have to come back."

(Third ignored hint – we always walked out with our usual goodie bag of drugs.)

Manhattan is 2.3 miles wide. It took more than an hour to travel that distance, wrong-way excursion not included. No way was I going to turn around and head back into the hornet's nest, especially having seen the 60-minute queue of cars at the inbound Lincoln Tunnel.

---

2 Most nurses carry enough supplies with them at all times to perform three-way, heart bypass surgery.

Negotiations ensued and it was agreed that 1) we were idiots albeit very tired ones and, 2) Sandra would call the prescriptions into our pharmacy, so we could go get them without driving back into Manhattan. Crisis avoided.

However, our great escape paled in comparison to Fariel's orgasm.

I have a knack for baking. I also have a knack for eating, so even though baking is somewhat therapeutic for me I'd resemble Orson Wells if I ate everything I made. I quickly developed the habit of taking most of what I bake elsewhere: the office, a friend's house, or family get-togethers. There was not a better group I could think of that deserved some homemade goodies than the staff at MSK. My staples are banana bread, chocolate chip cookies, snickerdoodles and brownies laced with caramel filled Dove chocolates. This last item has produced comments such as "What did you put in these, crack?" and "You are evil."

When I brought the brownies to the nurses, however, Fariel, a bombastic young lady pretty enough to conquer Bollywood and with enough personality for 20 people, had a different take that will remain in our treatment lore forever.

One day, our friends Rich and Jill had traveled to the city to visit Sally; personal visits always brightened both our days. The four of us sat in Sally's room chatting when suddenly Fariel burst in.

"Oh, my God," she said excitedly. "I just had some of your brownies. I think I came seven times." And then she walked out.

Following the brief pause of "Did she really just say that?" we all burst out laughing. I'm not sure she realized there were other people in the room, but, to her credit, she didn't care. That's who she is and we love her.

Regardless of our room assignment, Sally's bed represented an informal nurse break station, where they could hide from the chaos of the nurse bullpen and less than happy patients. We were a place where they could breathe and sit a spell. Much of the discussion with Kristyn, Fariel and Shirley concerned either the rigors of their continuing education or their upcoming weddings. I have learned through painful experience that when a group of women get together to discuss wedding plans, my help, and/or input, was not needed or for that matter even wanted.

Jasmine would visit and unload the stresses of raising a 13-year-old daughter, which speaks for itself.

"She's going to drive me crazy," Jasmine said one day after going through Sally's examination. After an outpouring of the latest pre-teen trauma, through which Sally listened patiently, as any good Freudian therapist would, Sally said, "She'll be fine. You're doing a great job with her. If she turns out like her Mom, you'll have nothing to worry about."

Veronica was either shaping up her handsome son to be presentable for the prom or was threatening to lock him in his room until his 30th birthday.

"That boy'll be the death of me," Veronica often muttered through her surgical mask, which she wore all through flu season.

Sally would always wave her off, "He'll be fine. He's got a strong Mom to guide him through it all."

By the sixth round of chemo, half the nursing staff instantly flocked to Sally's side before she could even get to the room and unpack; she had her own built-in welcoming committee. They all had to check in and see how Mom was doing.

We threw them all into apoplexy during one treatment when there was no space available on the seventh floor, so we were shipped to the fourteenth floor. Sally's nurses on seven were not about to sit still for that. Liz, Kristyn, Nick, and Shirley. made their way to 14 to check up on Sal and make sure everything was okay and to assure us they had the wheels in motion to bring us back "home.".

Within 6 hours we were back on the seventh floor.

By session six, Sally was starting to physically react to the chemo, feeling nauseous to the point of not eating. She was reaching her emotional limit on all things cancer and had slipped into a funk. One morning Kristyn, Alexa, and Fariel surprised Sal with a gift bag that had a good-sized mug with "Good Morning, Beautiful" printed on it. Not five minutes later Jasmine walked in with a teddy bear and a balloon. But they were not done. Petal P, who was Sal's nurse for one day - one day - came in to give hugs and sprinkle get-well fairy dust (metaphorically, I think) in the room.

During a subsequent treatment, the ladies of the house swarmed upon their star patient again, presenting her with a pair of full-size, pink boxing gloves, personally signed by the whole nursing crew.

Don't tell me nurses remain aloof to their patients.

One night as I walked through the corridor close to the change of shift, I saw a nurse named Fallon standing at the elevator, bundled in her parka, tears streaming down her face as she talked with Eleni, the nurse manager. Fallon was a pretty waif who looked like she was still in high school. She had never been assigned to Sally, but just from close proximity over time I learned most of the nursing staff by name. My heart ached; I wanted to give her a hug. I realized suddenly how fiercely protective I felt towards the nurses on seven, even the ones where no connection had been established. Several days later I passed Fallon in the corridor.

"Are you okay?" I asked, gently. She looked at me quizzically at first, and then she remembered.

"Oh. Yes. It was just a rough day."

"I'm sure those happen from time to time, especially on this floor."

She smiled and nodded, "They do, but I'm okay. That's sweet of you to ask."

Treatment timing worked in our favor, allowing us to make good on a threat to crash Kristyn's wedding. Sally donned her wig, and we made the trek to Staten Island. The ceremony was simple and beautiful, and Kristyn made a stunning bride. The highlight, however, was reaching the bride, groom, and mother of the bride in the receiving line.

"These are the Coopers," Kristyn said by way of introduction. Mom and Kristyn's husband lit up as if they were greeting old friends.

"Kristyn talks about you all the time," her mom said.

We felt as if we were instantly part of Kristyn's family from the start. Nurses are like that.

On the flip side, one night in the hospital, Sally and I sat half dozing when I realized there was a lot of commotion outside of the room. As I stuck my head in the hallway the intercom system screeched, "Code blue." Followed by a room number.

Nurses appeared from every direction, hitting the floor in crash cart mode, all heading for a room across the corridor. I stood and watched them work with a focused, calm urgency; in clockwork precision now that a patient's life was on the line.

Most of us approach our daily routines knowing what needs to be done within a fairly relaxed timeline. Nurses make life and death decisions within the span of seconds and with a level of intensity and professionalism second to none. As I watched them restore a critical patient, the non-critical nature of my job gave me a good right cross to the chops, emphasizing that on a scale of one to ten, where ten is the nursing profession, I concluded my job ranked at a negative 7,235 to the negative 1,127th power. This is a number so low that most online statistical calculators will be unable to complete the calculation, opting instead to implode in a cloud of smoke.

Other than nursing, there is no other profession that inspires, literally, thousands of posts on Pinterest and Facebook, with quotes about caring, compassion and not giving up. This one, however, remains the most telling:

"I'm a nurse and a Mom. Nothing scares me."

Names and contact info for the patient's nurses:

_____
_____
_____
_____
_____
_____
_____
_____
_____
_____
_____
_____

Things I can do to brighten a nurse or staff member's day:

_____
_____
_____
_____
_____
_____
_____

Notes:

Caregiver Tip #15

Be flexible. Allow for sudden unexpected shifts in the process. They will happen.

Some things will not always go the way you expect. Actually, none of this *really* goes the way you expect. Stay open to it all anyway. An army of doctors and other health professionals will send you down paths you never expected to be on. That's okay. Remember this was all new territory for everyone who came before you. You are not alone. Even when things feel out of control (which is, granted, most of the time) remain open to what you are experiencing.

Dr. G said, "I want to do a stem cell transplant."

He dropped a 50-megaton payload on us during the next post-chemo check-up.

"You are still about 85 to 90 percent clear," he said after reviewing the MRI results after the ninth chemo session. "I still want do one more as we discussed to see if we can knock out even more."

I felt all my muscles clench and my nerves about to snap. One additional chemo treatment had not provided any tangible results. I wanted to know why and what could be done about it. Deep inside I knew there was no answer to my first question and that Dr. G. was doing everything in his power to help Sally. Regardless, my internal pressure was reaching critical mass, but I held back the urge to scream.

Divorced from my own feelings, I saw much the same and more in Sally's face.

During treatments six, seven and eight, Sally was nauseous for 24-36 hours after the infusion and had to be coerced into eating anything during the entire stay. This wasn't fun anymore, if it ever really was.

I had to look around to see who just attached the car battery leads to my…well…neck. Spine-clenching fear grabbed me as hard as the original diagnosis.

Dr G. gave us all the valid medical reasons for the stem-cell transplant. "Here's the thought process: 1) you had a great reaction to chemo - no infections or other issues; 2) it avoids radiation and with brain lymphoma, unlike other cancers, there is no pinpointing the mass;[1] the entire brain gets radiated. The chances of the radiation causing permanent cognitive issues are higher the older the patient; and 3) we want to slam the door as hard as possible on the chance for relapsing. The transplant method, while not without risk of course, has proven the most effective without causing long term issues.

"I'm offering this as a possibility," he continued. "Next time you are in New York talk to Dr. Sauter. He's the expert and can give you all the details. Just think about it."

What was Sally's main concern? All together now...

"Can I keep my hair?"

Her hair had thinned significantly by this point, but she desperately wanted to hold onto what was left.

Dr. G. sighed thoughtfully, as he always does when giving unwanted answers, trying to quickly develop a positive spin.

"No," he said, "but the tradeoff is worth it if we can prevent any further relapse. Your hair will always grow back."

"What if it comes back grey or something weird," Sally said pouting.

I said, "Hey, grey hair is sexy." I could not have received a more evil look if I had said I was going to go home and shoot the dogs. Hey, I tried.

"Eighth floor, right?" I said to Dr. G.

"Eight or fourteen. It depends on where there's room." He must have sensed the worry and doubt we were feeling. "It's just something to think about. Talk to Dr. Sauter during your next treatment. He's a good guy."

During all the treatments on the seventh floor, I often climbed the stairs to the eighth floor to use the only decent sized bathroom I had found.

---

1 This was true at the time this was written but I am told is no longer the case. In fact most of the treatment reginment Sally experienced has changed radically in just eight years.

The eighth floor was the Bone Marrow Transplant (BMT) floor. In my mind, bone marrow transplants sounded painful and frightening. Again, the unknown. The patients on that floor, when mobile, shuffled through the halls in full mask and glove regalia, dragging an IV stand with at least a thousand different monitors regulating the same number of medications in IV bags. My heart went out to them, and I always said a small prayer of gratitude that our experience was less traumatic. Yet, there was a nagging little flame in the back of mind that nudged me just enough to let me know that our turn on the transplant floor was in the future. Naturally, I pushed that notion aside quickly. Now, it was staring me in the face.

Over the next three weeks we talked to anyone who would listen about the stem cell transplant. Our cheerleader Liz said "You can do this, no sweat." Naturally.

Nick, one of Sally's nurses, had gone through the process on the patient side.

"It sucks going through it," he said, "but it's completely worth it. It's like having the worst flu you can imagine, and you will be weak for a year or so afterward. Everyone on the eighth floor knows what they are doing and will be with you every step of the way."

"So, in the long run, it's the way to go?" I asked.

"No question."

We acquiesced to a meeting with Dr. Sauter, the stem cell guru, who looked like your standard soap opera actor-doctor: Tall, fit, sandy haired, black rimmed glasses, millennial George Michael beard.

"I talked with Dr. Gavrilovic. He said you were a prime candidate for a stem cell transplant." He had a soft, confident tone. I imagined he was eyeing us as the new test subjects for whatever this whole transplant deal entailed. We listened to his pitch.

"Look, the process will be uncomfortable for a few days, but we have the staff and the medications to get you through it. The success rate we've been seeing is great. It avoids radiation, which is the big thing, and the patients who have gone through it have great track records of significantly less relapsing than those who don't do it or choose radiation."

The bottom line was that even though our fears were clearly on the surface, anything was better than radiation; Sally fit into an age demographic where the risks of permanent brain damage from radiation were higher than someone half her age. Plus, anything we could do to reduce the chances of a relapse was worth it.

We'd come this far putting ourselves in MSK's hands. We decided to go forward with the procedure.

Up until this point, Sally had been biting the bullet by using an IV pic line in her arm with all the infusions rather than having a port grafted to her body. Having tubes temporarily implanted in her chest was not something she was ready to deal with. With the transplant, she would have no choice. A port would be installed, and, in the end, would become a double-edged sword.

May first was port installation day. Sally had not been allowed to eat or drink since the night before. We had to be at Sloan by nine in the morning for testing to ensure Sally's body could handle it. The procedure was scheduled for two that afternoon, following which Sally could ingest some nourishment.

By five in the afternoon, we were still waiting. I still don't know how Sally was putting up with not eating or drinking for nearly 24 hours. I would have bludgeoned someone with an IV stand. At six o'clock they finally wheeled her away and by eight that night Sally was in recovery and coming out of the anesthesia with two nifty white tubes about six inches long sticking out of her chest, dangling above her right boob. I thought maybe it would catch on as a fashion accessory in goth or steampunk circles.

The next step, scheduled for May 12th was the harvesting of Sally's stem cells, to be frozen for the duration and thawed once she was ready for the transplant, so we had time to rejuvenate our stamina and mentally prepare. Or so we thought.

Ten days later, the ground vanished from under our feet.

Things I can do when unexpected changes occur:

_____
_____
_____
_____
_____
_____
_____
_____
_____
_____
_____
_____
_____

People/Professionals I can call when overwhelmed:

_____
_____
_____
_____
_____
_____
_____
_____

Notes:

Caregiver Tip #16

Bad days happen.
Remember, they don't last forever. Focus on taking one step at a time and trust tomorrow will be better.

The patient will have bad days.
YOU will have bad days.
It's all part of the new normal. Little things may help for the patient - some flowers, a visit from a member of the family or friends, an ice cream cone. Bad days don't last forever - and there is always help available for the patient...

and the caregiver.

When the caregiver has a bad day, the first reaction is to brush it off and feel guilty - "I'm not the patient. How dare I have a bad day?"
You Are Allowed To Have Bad Days. And you will. That spirituality discussed earlier? It comes in pretty handy when things are not going well....

I heard the scream. Then what sounded like a pile of logs crashed on the floor.

I was sitting on the bed tying my shoes. May 11th. We were in limbo between the last chemo treatment and the scheduled stem cell transplant and life was semi-normal. I had started going back to the office a couple days a week; Sally was taking it slow around the house, each of us was mentally gearing up for the impending, month-long transplant hospital stay.

I jumped off the bed and flew across the hall to find Sally splayed on the bathroom floor, face up, eyes open, dazed and muttering, "I'm fine. I'm fine." A sure sign that she was anything but fine.

"What happened? Did you hit your head on anything?" The woman was in La-La Land and I'm firing questions like a magpie.

"No. I'm fine. I'm fine," she said starting to get up. I gently grabbed her shoulder and pushed her back to the floor.

"Just hang here a second. Stay put." Any competent EMS person would check the eyes for concussion and the head for contusions. EMS material I am not. I made neither examination. I just wanted her to lie still so I could collect my wits. After a minute I caught my breath and helped her slowly to her feet.

Immediately, blood started flowing from her nose.

I grew up with a neighborhood kid whose nose bled if a falling leaf brushed past his head. His mom always made him sit in a chair with his head tilted back. That's the extent of my medical training when it came to nosebleeds. I got Sally back in bed with a pillow under her neck to keep her head back. After a few minutes and the better part of a box of blood-soaked Kleenex disposed of, I asked, "What happened?"

"I was brushing my teeth and leaned over to spit. That's the last thing I remember."

"Did you hit your head on the sink or the tub?"

"No. I just crumbled to the floor I guess."

I didn't buy this completely as I distinctly heard her scream "OW." Our bathroom is smaller than a walk-in closet for Mini-Me. We lived in an old farmhouse built in the late 1800's and while the bathtub was Munchkin sized, it was an older one made of enameled steel. My main concern was that she fell backwards and hit her head on it. Gently probing the back of her head, Sally said she wasn't hurting anywhere, that her head felt fine. Her nose, however, would not stop bleeding.

The scope of my diagnostic capabilities exhausted, I sent for the cavalry. Two phone calls to Sloan Kettering later, we were on our way to our third home, the ER at Princeton Medical Center.

While I went through the morning's events with the ER admitting staff, Sally presented an interesting tableau in the waiting room, stretched prone on the familiar Pepto-Bismol pink vinyl bench, her nose sporting half a roll of semi-bloody toilet paper.

The admissions nurse summoned Sally in order to go through the initial triage, saying, "Let me get you a wheelchair."

Sally, never wanting to trouble anyone, jumped up and waved her off. "I don't need a wheelchair."

"Take the damn wheelchair," I said sitting her back on the bench. There are times when the caregiver is required to issue direct commands. My gut told me this was one of them.

I wheeled her into the triage office and within ten seconds, Sally turned to me, eyes wide and swimming, and said, "I'm going to faint," and then proceeded to do just that, her head flopping back on the chair like stone, her mouth and eyes wide open.

Good God, she's dead, I thought, as the only other time I saw that expression on someone's face was my mom's face the day she died. The fear and anxiety I experienced on the journey thus far was a romp with Mary Poppins in a chalk sidewalk painting in comparison what I now felt; I was in a place of fear I never knew existed, paralyzed beyond the ability to act.

Fortunately, the triage attendant knew her stuff. She immediately slapped an icepack on Sally's stretched neck, jammed the wheelchair into fourth gear and beat Usain Bolt's 100-meter dash record as she raced Sally through the ER with me bringing up the rear amidst whispered comments from bystanders of ,"What's going on?" and "I wonder what happened."

Just get out of the way rubberneckers, I wanted to scream. But didn't.

ER nurses quickly flocked into the curtained cubicle in which Sally was parked. That magic nurse mojo must have kicked in as Sally's eyelids fluttered and she slowly raised her head. The professionals scurried around Sally slapping on a blood pressure cuff and firing off questions. "What's your name? What day is it? Where are you?"

Sally groggily responded with the correct answers. I stood on the edges of the activity and attempted to lower my blood pressure into numbers without commas.

Over the next couple hours Sally repeatedly told her tale that she just passed out at home but didn't hit her head on anything. Additional examinations by the hospital staff confirmed the absence of a concussion or fractures. They shifted into heavier-duty, blood absorption methods, switching from Kleenex to sterile, waffle-sized hospital gauze pads. Regardless, the blood flow continued. She was also spiking a three-digit fever; an even bigger clue that something was amiss.

By late morning, Sally had been admitted. Her nose was still bleeding, the culprit pinpointed on a platelet level of 40, far from the normal range of 160 to 400. Once she was transferred to a regular room, a course of IV platelets was administered. Now it was a waiting game, hoping the transfusion would boost Sally's platelet level and that her body's natural defenses would kick in to staunch the blood flow. "Regular room" in this case was defined as a standard, hospital-sized room but set up with a single bed and a windowed nurse monitoring station attached to it.

As if the morning's activities had not been enough, and in what must surely have been a case of God hitting the Jack Daniel's bottle, this was the day our son Stephen picked to pay a visit to his mother. Understand this, Stephen is the sensitive artist and in his eyes, you don't fuck with his mother. In his early teens, in between practicing with his punk band Censored Society and creating works of art on his bedroom wall, he used to yell at guys in Shop-Rite who, in his opinion, let their eyes wander a tad too long in his mothers direction. Stephen has never minced words his entire life, whether it was through genuine empathy or as the onset of a more direct verbal assault. For the most part, this has stood him in good stead. It's also created some conflicts of opinion with his friends and sometimes with total strangers who felt it necessary to drive their opposing logic home in a more physical manner. But that's a different ER story.

Fortunately, Stephen appeared after Sally was moved to a room and thankfully, he missed the ER chaos. He sat at the foot of her bed, his face a mask of frustration. This was his mom and being helpless did not sit well.

"I'm angry," he said without shifting his eyes from his sleeping Mother, a wad of deepening red cotton shoved up the right side of her nose.

I replied, "I understand. Not that it's helpful, but this is the worst this journey has been. Up until now it's been sort of a breeze. She'll be okay." I'm not sure which one of us I was attempting to convince.

The young doctor running the show, a Patton Oswalt-looking guy who had a similar sense of humor, beckoned me into the hallway. I grabbed Stephen's shoulder as reassuringly as I could and left him to process the day's events.

"Listen," the doctor said, "we are a great community hospital, but given what she's gone through and is still going through, she needs to be back at Sloan to make sure everything is okay. My assumption is the drop in platelet levels and blood counts is due to her last chemo treatment. We don't want to jeopardize the work that she's done thus far, and we are not equipped to specialize in her disease."

I heartily agreed. Even though they had taken every precaution, getting her back to Sloan was the first priority.

How that was going to happen was up in the air. I wasn't sure where exactly to start or who to call to set this all in motion. The stem cell team's jurisdiction had not officially kicked in at this point, and Dr. G. was not immediately reachable. So, I did what anyone else would do in this situation.

I sent text messages to Sally's crew of Sloan nurses.

All of them responded, which by this point should not have surprised me; when their star patient is in need, they move. Jasmine was the first to respond even though she had recently transferred to a different unit and location within the Sloan system. It didn't matter. This was her surrogate Mom.

"How do I go about setting up an ambulance ride for her highness," I said to Jasmine after we had exchanged phone numbers via text, and I explained the situation to her.

"I know we've done it before. Let me make some phone calls and find out." Based on Jasmine's efforts, the right people in Princeton spoke with the right people in New York; the ride was scheduled for the following day, subject to Sally's blood levels recovering.

Worried, but with the knowledge that his mom was being cared for on a number of different fronts, Stephen left that afternoon with a promise from me to keep him in the loop.

From the window ledge of Sally's fifth floor southwest-facing room, I watched the sun descend on the newly budded trees; all the new spring-green deepened in the orange glow of the sunset. Sally continued to sleep, and I took a moment to breathe in the quiet. On reflection, days of panic and chaos fly by like Christmas Day. We had covered a lot of ground in 12 hours, and I was able to let go, now that a plan was in place. Amidst my silent notions of gratitude for the continuing level of care we were receiving, was the hope that Sally would improve quickly. I sat long enough to see the sun disappear and some stars ignite in the sky.

Sally awoke when the nurse came in to take vitals.

"I'm going to head home and deal with the dogs, get some food and some sleep. You okay on your own? I can come back if you want."

She gently shook her head. "No. Go. Get something to eat." After a kiss and squeeze of her hand, I headed home.

The next day, I was holding my breath as I entered Sally's room, only to find her propped up in bed, TV blaring, and without any red rags hanging from her nose. She was still white as a ghost, but at least the bleeding had stopped.

"The numbers are up," she said, smiling, referring to her platelet and red blood counts. While I was ecstatic with the news, I couldn't help notice the start of not one but two deep purple bruises forming under each eye. I sat on the bed with what I'm sure was a self-satisfied smirk on my puss.

"Didn't hit anything going down, eh?" I said.

"Well???" she said with the smile of a kid caught with her hand in the cookie jar.

What was apparent, even to the Queen of Denial, was that she most certainly slammed her face on the bathroom sink when she passed out.

"Everyone is going to think this is all bullshit and that I punched you in the nose."

It took the better part of the day, but by mid-afternoon, Cinderella's Ambulance had arrived in Princeton with driver and attendant, who was a short, brassy woman, late 40's early 50's, whom I liked immediately. We passed a break station in the hospital on the way to Sally's room and she grabbed a can of Coke and slipped it into her pocket. "Gotta take it where I can get it," she said. Just from talking to her, I knew she had back stories that were funny and tough. She would not take crap from anyone.

I was bummed that I didn't get to ride in the ambulance, but logistically we needed our car in New York, thinking Sally would be a day or two in-patient before we could go home. Relieved that we were headed back to our familiar "beach house" in Manhattan, I waved them good-bye as the ambulance pulled away and went home to throw some clothes in a bag for both of us.

A few hours later I found Sally in an isolated room at MSK and noticed a business card from the EMS attendant, with all her personal information scribbled on the back. On the ride, she and Sally had bonded, swapped life stories and were planning to get together after all this was over. Someday I'll stopped being surprised by shit like this — only Sally.

"They were waiting for me," she said with a smile. "They wheeled me out of the ambulance and everyone in Urgent Care was Mrs. Cooper this, Mrs. Cooper that."

"Sometimes you want to go where everybody knows your name…"

To say we were "home" may be derivative, but it's still the truth. The change in Sally just being at Sloan was 180 degrees. She had color in her face for the first time since passing out and her temperature was back to normal.

The room's western exposure afforded a wonderful view of sunsets bouncing off the steel and glass towers of the east side, and having no roommate was an added bonus. But that's where the bonuses ended.

Sometime after blood cultures had been drawn, a doctor I didn't know entered the room. "Hi. I'm one of the infectious disease doctors."

That alone sent alarm bells clanging in my head.

He continued, "You've developed a staph infection, which is probably the reason your blood levels became so low. We're going to start you on a full course of antibiotics." Sounded reasonable to me. "Also, just to be on the safe side, we are going to remove your port. Many times that's the source of these types of infections."

It dawned on me that we had just shifted into a longer-than-two-day-stay mode.

"What's the timing of all this?" I said.

"We're going to remove the port tonight. Hopefully, the antibiotics will kick out the infection quickly, and we can install a new port by Friday. After that we can send you home." Sally's face sagged, clearly reflecting the huge emotional letdown she felt.

"Aw shit," I said.

"Tell me about it," Sally said nodding in agreement.

"You know what else this means?"

She stared at me, wheels spinning in her head.

"We're not going to able to crash Fariel's wedding." The ceremony was set for the upcoming Saturday.

"Maybe, maybe not. When we get out on Friday we'll ask if we can still go."

Han Solo popped into my head:

"I have a bad feeling about this."

Restricted from wandering around until her blood levels became more robust and the antibiotics had a chance to start beating the crap out of the staph germs, we spent our time in the room napping, eating and watching television, which was fine for the first 24 hours. Restlessness and boredom quickly set in. Sitting around the hospital for no reason didn't sit well with the White Tornado, she had things to do and sitting in bed, even on the weekends, has never been part of her nature.

In December of 1989, we both contracted viral pneumonia, not much fun as Christmas approached with eight- and six-year-olds in the house. I took to bed right after Thanksgiving and virtually never left until the first week of February. Sally would sleep, then get up and do stuff. Twenty minutes up, twenty back in bed. Trying to get her to let herself be sick was worth my life. She had her own recovery schedule and that was that.

This sitting around the hospital stuff wasn't going to fly, but she had no choice.

Sally's mood worsened with each passing hour in isolation. As a caregiver, I was wracking my brain trying to come up with something to lighten things up. Our daughter, Beth, came to the rescue. She called me and wanted to visit, as the last time she saw her mother was in Princeton with a bloody gauze rag stuffed up her nose. I didn't let Sally know about the arrangements and the next day I led Beth into the room announcing, "Look who I found."

Sally's face completely brightened up. Her baby had come to see her. They spent a couple hours just gabbing, but it was enough to put a smile back on Sally's face and release some of the pressure I was feeling.

Based on what the doctors and nurses were telling us, we were gearing up for a Friday release. This was the first week that time dragged slower than a two-legged turtle in molasses. We knew that two things had to happen before we were discharged: The infection needed to recede, and a new port needed to be inserted into Sally's chest. By Thursday, neither of these had come to pass. Sally, however, was still focused on leaving Friday. I could see the train of disappointment coming around the bend.

Late Friday afternoon, Dr. Infectious Disease[1] paid a visit with the final proclamation.

"The infection has subsided, but it will be Monday before the port can be re-installed. After that we can get you out of here."

Once the doctor left, Sally broke down sobbing. I sat on the bed holding her, neither of us saying as word. To say she had slammed into the tolerance wall and was heartbroken falls short of the mark. Aside from missing Fariel's wedding, this little bump impacted the stem cell transplant dates. We had mentally geared up to be through the process by sometime in June; we were now looking at July.

One full year from the beach party that was the start of this journey.

As it turned out, Sally did not get re-ported until late Monday, so it was Tuesday before we were released. Eight days of unplanned hospitalization

---

1 I never did learn his name. By this point, I needed a Playbill in order to keep track of all the players in this production.

between Princeton and MSK. We didn't leave MSK with the usual chemo bag of pharmaceutical goodies, but, like parting contestants on a game show, we didn't leave empty handed.

In fact, once we settled back home, one corner of our bedroom was transformed into Medical Supplies 'R' Us: boxes stacked on boxes holding surgical gloves, alcohol wipes, surgical masks, port caps, 9-volt batteries....

Yes. Batteries.

Dr. Infectious Disease prescribed continued antibiotic treatment for a couple weeks as a precautionary move in order to ensure all the staph squigglies were wiped out. This required Sally to carry a battery-driven pump, 24-hours a day, which could be programmed to introduce the medicine into her body in specific doses and set intervals.

Small, clear I.V. bags held the medication and the square transistor radio batteries, the ones we pressed on our tongues to verify the childhood myth concerning cool electric shocks. Both required a daily change. Given the nine-volt power source, I wasn't surprised the pump itself resembled a steroid overloaded transistor radio, but with a touchpad controlling a menu-driven application, not unlike programming a thermostat. The pump attached via Velcro inside a canvas case along with the bag of medication. The sling-like apparatus, complete with shoulder strap, sported clear plastic tentacles that were hooked up to the new ports embedded in Sally's chest.[2]

The patient probably could handle the required daily maintenance, but the risk of infection decreased if they didn't, so my caregiving skills had to expand further. One more thing on the plate.

In addition to the daily battery and med bag replacement, every five days the entire apparatus needed cleaning and sterilizing, inside and out.

---

[2] I've mentioned it previously, but I get astounded when I stop and realize that somebody had to think of this rig, and then prove it actually worked.

A visiting nurse paid a visit to our house to instruct me on the proper technique, one that did not endanger the patient.

She explained the process and then said. "Okay. You do it."

"You mean 'do it' do it, or just explain it?" I said sheepishly.

"Do it do it."

Donning surgical gloves and armed with mounds of surgical wipes, I sterilized the ports, installed new port caps, and replaced the sterilized, heavy-gauge, saran wrap glued to Sally's chest over the port entry using special adhesive removal junk that prevented instant skin removal. Next the port lines had to be flushed by a sterile saline solution in a syringe that hooked up to the port line.

Happily, I passed the hands-on exam.

Confidentially, I looked forward to this procedure not just for the gadget tinkering pleasure it gave or the good feeling I got from doing something tangible, but also for its base, carnal potential. To say that our sex life was reduced to a non-existent state should be obvious given everything that was happening. I showed Sally the hospital-provided pamphlet entitled "Sex After Treatment," but she just laughed. The thoughts I was having were conspicuously absent from the literature anyway. Sally's port entry was about four inches above her right boob. As the Sterilization Day process was easiest for Sally sans shirt or bra, I looked forward with lecherous glee to seeing her boobs every five days or so. I felt like a seventh grader having fantasies during math class of the Playboy bunnies in the magazine hidden under his mattress at home. Cheap thrills? You bet.

I'd be midway through the process and Sally would say, "What the hell are you smiling at?"

I did tell her what was going through my mind and received the appropriate eye-rolling response so please save your energy if you were thinking of firing off any scathing, feminist hate-mail. It is my wife for God's sake.

Sally learned to sleep with the pump bag, cuddling it as if Pooh Bear had crawled into her arms. Every so often I heard the pump kick on with a soft whirring sound, signaling the flow of medication. I lay in bed with jealous thoughts swirling in my head. Why can't I have my own rig supplying, oh, Ativan, Lunesta or even some Knob Creek Bourbon? Nonetheless, the immediate crisis had passed, and we'd survived more than one bad day in the process.

But a few more waited in the wings.

Imagine the worst bout of the flu you've ever had. Now imagine being run over by a double decker bus. For the patient, that's what surviving the stem cell protocol is all about. If I hadn't known this was part of the deal, I would have been thoroughly heartbroken watching Sally, barely able to lift her head off the pillow. We experienced this invalid stage, even though our star stem-cell nurse, Elisabetta, a dark curly haired and olive skinned Major General, seemingly born out of a chromosome dance between Debra Winger and Sal Mineo, insisted Sally get on her feet and move around the room, and eat something. Sally couldn't leave the room while her white counts were still at zero, but Elisabetta wanted to see some motion out of her.

Caregivers have to deal with all things scary and all things gross and disgusting (vomiting foot long esophageal scabs, listening to roommates manage sputum accumulation). Fortunately, the nurses are there to handle the really icky parts.

One of the by-products of the full week of chemo is the possibility of some of the tenderer and mucus-like membranes in Sally's body getting burned, not an uncommon occurrence when dealing with chemo or radiation. The only pain Sally experienced post-chemo was a sore throat, making swallowing a chore. If nothing else, the hospital was all about managing pain and discomfort so on Sunday the 28th, a painkiller was added to the myriad of bags already hanging from Sally's IV stand.

Sunday remained quiet, as Sundays usually do in the hospital. My biggest issue of the day was what I would do for dinner as the cafeteria closes at three on the Sabbath. Inevitably, I wound up at Lunetta's Pizza for two slices of the best mushroom pepperoni pizza in Manhattan. Barely wide enough for a counter and a single row of tables, I snagged a table near the front window and watched the east side of Manhattan fly by as I gleefully bit into the gooey cheeziness of pepperoni and mushrooms. At this point searing the inside of my mouth to shreds didn't matter.

Sated by gluttony, I strolled north on First Avenue, a golden sun dipping in the west to cast skyscraper shadows in random stripes across the east side. By this time, I was thoroughly comfortable walking around a twenty street, four avenue area of the city that really did feel like a second home. It is simple to feel that way when there is no New York rent or taxes to pay, not to mention (semi) free room and board and an entire recreation center at my disposal. In Manhattan, living and visiting are disparate states of consciousness.

Back in the room as evening settled in, Sally and I were quietly talking, her throat still on the rough side, about what was going on in the world.

She started to say, "What did you have for…" and then stopped, staring at me as if everything went blank.

"Dinner?" I asked.

She nodded and I told her about my Lunetta's feast, trying desperately not to reveal the Queen Mother of knots slamming into my guts. We talked further and two more blank spots in her speech happened, the same blank spots that happened at the start of all of this, the same blank spots in her speech from a year ago, the same helpless look in her eyes when she could not articulate a thought. Panic coursed through me…what the hell was going on?

I sat her up and, purposefully, gave her a cup of water to hold so I could surreptitiously watch her hands for tremors and to see if she held on to it. She didn't drop it, but I could see her fingers wobbling, as if under remote control from an unknown source.

My God. Here we are at the end of the treatment road, and it looks like we are right back where we started. Did the stem cell chemo cause permanent damage? Was everything she endured over the past 12 months all for nothing? To say I was frightened was an understatement. This was not supposed to happen.

As nonchalantly as possible, I left the room and tracked down her nurse, expressing my observations and concerns. The nurse came in to talk to Sally to make her own observations and told me she would contact the doctor on duty.

Sally was back asleep, and I was left to ride out my internal storm; the nurse told me the team would be in first thing Monday morning to see what was up. Swell.

That night lasted forever, as I sat on the sofa looking south at the lights of the Ed Koch bridge and the apartment buildings in between. The one-sided conversation with my Higher Power went something like this:

"Hey. This is all yours. I'm giving up control to you, with at least the modicum of faith that I can muster that this will all be okay. I am beyond grateful for everything that has happened thus far. Please keep an eye out on Sally and all the doctors and nurses under her care. This is out of my hands. I'm counting on you."

Dawn was forever in coming, but finally the sky brightened over Roosevelt Island, the sun making the candy cane striped chimney stacks across the river gleam as if lit on a Christmas tree. Finally, the white-coated herd flooded into the room to check on Sally.

Throughout this whole experience, there was always "a team," six to ten people who enter the room each morning with the doctor and nurse coordinator on duty to check on the patient. It's kind of funny to watch because as they do their rounds, they huddle in the hallway between rooms, holding impromptu updates and discussing patient treatment options, a wall of white lab coats in a strategy huddle.

I sat on the couch, bleary-eyed from a sleepless night, while they circled the bed as if preparing to provide last rites. Due to Sally's speech issue, I once again found myself as chief status spokesperson. The doctor in charge that day, a tall woman I had never seen before, who reminded me of Pippi Longstocking with the same curly red tresses but worn down instead of in pigtails and a manner somewhere between ah-shucks Andy Griffith and Joan Rivers, quickly diagnosed the issue.

She said, with a smile, "The pain medication she is getting is morphine-based. It's strong enough that when it hits the areas of weakness in her brain, the places where the lymphoma clouds appeared, it will produce behavior not unlike the quirks Sally had prior to treatment. We will switch medications and she'll be fine."

I wanted to cry with relief. The best thing that happened, continually, as a caregiver was being with staff who explained everything in layman's detail.

The medication switch was made as promised and, to my extreme joy, within 12 hours Sally was back to thinking and speaking.

I needed a drink.

When bad days happen I will:

Notes:

Caregiver Tip #17

Help other caregivers.
Listen. Share your experience.

Share your experiences with others - especially those who are new, sporting that "deer in the headlights" look. They will feel better talking to someone who has been there; the best thing you can do is just listen. As a bonus, you will feel better just by helping someone in need and also talking about your journey.

It's a caregiver duality, not unlike any good Twelve Step mantra:

You can't keep it, if you don't give it away.

"I'm exhausted," I said, in response to Nancy G.'s inquiry concerning my state of mind. I don't have a rational explanation why I chose that moment to forego the hackneyed "I'm fine" cover story and express the tiniest of true feeling. Perhaps it was the appearance of a high school friend, absent from my life for 40 years, making the effort to visit Sally in the hospital, or the fact that she had recently been in the caregiver role with her husband Fred and could read my inner weariness, having just trudged through the same experience.

"I know," she said. "It's part of the deal and you'll feel that way for awhile. Take some breaks and try to get more sleep."

"Oh, yeah right," I said, darkly chuckling. "Sleep…"

"I know, I know. Especially here in the hospital. I get it. But you have to keep yourself healthy. If you get sick, it won't help either of you. And don't feel like you have to do everything. Call me if you need anything or even if you want to just talk."

After hugging her and packing her off on the elevator, I felt oddly reinforced, having unwittingly stumbled upon something brand new; a caregiver resource. It was April 2015 and after five months of treatments, taking care of myself was a new concept as everything else thus far was geared toward Sally's treatment. Perhaps the lessons I needed were sinking in with greater ease than they had at the start of the journey. It became obvious this particular lesson took up residence in my consciousness on the day I was able to offer it to another weary caregiver.

Sally and I lounged in her room one day, waiting impatiently for the blood counts to come back when a nurse we didn't recognize entered Sally's room and said, "Hi Mrs. Cooperman."

We looked at each other blankly. "Ummm, no," I said. "We're the Coopers." The nurse looked perplexed and silently left, we assumed to check her records again.

"Think someone screwed up?" Sally asked.

"Dunno."

But that was the last we heard of whatever was going on until….

The next day when a different nurse repeated the same song and dance, greeting Sally as Mrs. Cooperman.

By the third day, after a repeat performance, I had to find out what was going on. Maybe Sally's records were wrong and that certainly needed addressing.

Kristyn was busy at the computer in the nurses' station but jumped up when she saw me loitering outside the door.

"What's up?"

I explained the Cooperman/Cooper deal we had witnessed over the past few days.

Kristyn smiled wryly. "Yeah. There is a Mrs. Cooperman. You guys are confusing everyone."

Mrs. Cooperman just happened to be on the same treatment schedule as Mrs. Cooper, and the two of them were playing havoc with the newbie nurses on the floor. To add additional Marx Brothers insanity, the current treatment had them camped out in adjoining rooms. Thank God they were never roommates; it would have been ugly to see the nursing staff strewn in the hallway after committing mass hari-kari.

I approached Mrs. Cooperman's room and knocked on the door.

"I'm one of the Coopers. Are you seeing the same nurse confusion that we are?"

The two women in the room chuckled and nodded, "Oh yes."

In the bed was an older woman sitting up, also attached to several IV lines. Next to her sat a young woman I correctly assumed was Mrs. Cooperman's daughter. I had previously seen her on the floor, and we had said passing "Hi's" but had never spoken.

Through subsequent conversations, as there was always at least a two-day overlap in their treatment schedules, I discovered that the daughter, Abby, was from Switzerland; she had left husband and children at home, and had traveled to the US to be a full-time caretaker for her mom. Had I been completely separated from family for months and been on call twenty-four seven, I would have graced the East Side of Manhattan with a King Kong jack-knife off the Chrysler Building.

During a later treatment as I walked down the hospital corridor, I spotted Abby leaning against the wall outside her mom's room, head down, eyes cast on the floor. As I approached, I recognized her expression, one of crashing head-first into the stress-wall; that "I cannot take one more minute of this" look that all caretakers get occasionally. Had the wall crumbled behind her, she would have crumbled with it. I stopped in front of her, and she looked at me; even behind the thick round glasses I could see tears welling in front of the lost expression. I barely knew the woman, but I took her in my arms while she collapsed into sobs.

After the tsunami passed, I said, "What's going on?"

"I'm sorry. I feel foolish. Nothing is going on."

"You've just had enough."

"Yeah," she said, quietly awed at my recognition of her feelings.

"Don't kid yourself, being a caretaker is tough stuff – sometimes just as hard as being a patient. You've got nothing to be sorry about. I had a meltdown a couple weeks ago; totally lost it screaming at my boss over the phone. I'm surprised I still have a job. I never saw it coming, it was just… there"

She sighed heavily, gathering herself together. "I know, but I really feel…"

"Guilty."

"Yeah. That's it. Like I'm not supposed to feel this way. I'm not the one with cancer, you know?"

"Even Superman morphed into Clark Kent from time to time."

At least I got the inklings of a smile out of her.

Throughout treatment we naturally fell into being co-caregiver resources, checking in from time to time, even if both of us felt strong. Knowing an experienced resource is available was half the battle to keeping our sanity.

Names and contact info of other caregivers:

_____
_____
_____
_____
_____
_____
_____
_____
_____
_____
_____
_____
_____

Ways I can help other caregivers:

_____
_____
_____
_____
_____
_____
_____
_____

Notes:

Caregiver Tip #18

Don't shy away from conversations about death and dying.

It is, unfortunately, still part of the cancer world. People still die from it. There is always the specter of death running through the patient's and caregiver's minds. Some patients have to face the prospect head on. It's better to have the hard conversations out in the open than leaving it unspoken. Caregiver resources are beginning to crop up everywhere (see *Appendix A: Caregiver Resources*). On one level, talk about it when someone you know succumbs. On another level, have the conversation when death is not staring anyone in the face.

You're not alone.

Over the years my overblown cynicism had led me to wondering, with all the money donated to cancer research, why haven't they come up with a cure yet? Now that we have become statistics in the ongoing battle, I get it. In my ignorant mind, the word "cancer" was the same as saying "measles" or "polio," a single word representing a single condition, a single cause and therefore, a single solution. Only now that we were immersed into the world of this disease did I learn of its devious nature. Discovering a cure is like nailing Jello to a tree. Cancer constantly mutates, so every time a treatment is developed that shows promise in stopping a certain type of cancer growth, and there are literally thousands of different types, cancer finds a way to alter itself around any medical roadblocks and continue its destructive path in a totally new form. In the ongoing battle, research has progressed to the point where cancer is starting to be treated on a genetic level. Soon each patient will be able to get a customized treatment based on their unique DNA.

Nonetheless, cancer is a mean bitch. Even though we were pushing through the treatment phase and had met so many beautiful roommates, nurses, doctors and hospital staff, death appeared consistently to remind us of what Yasminda, one of Sally's nurses, expressed so eloquently in a social media post:

> *"When your 39 y/o patient dies and you have to look at his wife and kids at his bedside, when you've spent months caring for them, watching him fade away, when you just want to scream "why??" when you can't stop crying because life is so valuable and delicate and under appreciated.....*
>
> *I just want to go home and curl up in a little ball, cuddled up with my children and husband. Because cancer sucks! Because cancer doesn't discriminate- young, old, black, white, rich or poor.*
> *Because in a heartbeat we can all be gone."*

All life is fragile and at any moment anything can change, regardless of the expertise, care and medical advances.

Somehow worrying about paying the gas bill, the latest political struggle at work, getting the grass mowed, government insanity, changing the oil in the car, etc., all dropped out of the top 100 things that matter in life. Time became more precious than I could ever have imagined.

Discussions about death between caregiver and patient are inevitable, especially when the Grim Reaper visited close to home. More often than not, the first instance of discussing mortality arises when the hospital staff presents patients with advanced directive forms.

As Sally signed the form naming me as the decision maker she said, "I'm not going anywhere you know. I have things left to do."

"I've always told you that you're going to outlive me," I said. I use humor to deflect from dealing with uncomfortable feelings. I can suck it up and have serious conversations, especially when Sally calls me on my shit, but my natural tendency from years of childhood training was flight, not fight. For this reason, I never asked Sally directly how she felt about the possibility of dying. It was a conversation I wasn't ready to have this early in the game.

Ready or not, though, death can and will pay a visit.

On June 8th, Sally learned that her first Sloan roommate, Kathie, had passed away in December about a week after we left the hospital. We were saddened and surprised as she appeared to be bouncing back so well. While we mourned her passing, we were grateful of having met her, being able to share a brief visit on the mortal plane.

Death doesn't play favorites, and caregivers are not immune.

Of the handful of people on the planet with whom I have a true soul connection, my friend Rose was near the top of the list. Aside from being the ultimate Italian Mama, Rose, her husband Pete and their kids opened their homes to us when we traveled to Florida. Pete was "the mayor" of Anna Maria Island. Not literally, but he was one of those guys everyone knew and liked with personality for five people and a willingness to be there for others.

During the course of Sally's treatment, I got a call from Rose; Pete was diagnosed with cancer just about everywhere. It was a massive stage four attack that took him quickly, in retrospect, but agonizingly slow for Rose who was stumbling down the caregiver road looking for miracles with grasping hands. She reached out to Sally and me, lost in the pain of watching Pete suffer and knowing she was going to lose the love of her life, her partner in everything, and was staring down the reality of being alone in the world. Her sense of helplessness was far beyond anything I had yet experienced, and just being available for her was all I could do. The weather had turned warm in Manhattan, and I spent a lot of time in St. Catherine's park, just listening to Rose on the phone. Being a silent ear is the single most important aspect of caregiving. I related to her feelings of helplessness and fear when I could, but more than anything I just wanted to give her a safe place to talk, scream and cry. I was not surprised to learn the biggest weight Rose was carrying was fear concerning how her kids would react. I spent most of my time reminding her to take care of herself while she worried about everyone else. Self-neglect is the number one issue on the caretakers hit parade.

When Pete died, Rose felt the inevitable mix of fear, sadness, and relief. What hurt her the most, however, was the guilt she felt for feeling relieved that Pete had passed away, an all-too-common reaction with caregivers losing a patient or loved one. An enormous caretaker burden is lifted yet we don't give ourselves permission to feel that relief without guilt. How dare we feel relieved when someone we love dies? It didn't make any sense, but I heard over and over from caregivers that guilt weighed heavily on their souls. Rose's feelings were raw and would remain that way for some time.

After Pete's passing, Rose attempted to build some semblance of a new life. She moved from Tennessee to Colorado to be closer to her grown children, she contacted grief support groups, and sought employment in her new location. She put on a brave face, but she lost a lot of weight, and every time we spoke the pain and sadness was palpable in her voice.

Eventually, Rose decided to move back to Tennessee. I'm not sure why. Maybe to get some closure or maybe she was still in flight mode. A couple months passed where we didn't connect on the phone and I had a nagging thought that I needed to call her, a thought I knew better than to ignore. But I did.

One day Sally tracked me down in the kitchen at home.

"What's going on with Rose?" she asked, a mixture of shock and fear on her face.

"What are you talking about?"

Sally showed me a social media post asking for prayers for Rose. She had suffered a brain aneurysm and a heart attack.

Within five days, she was gone.

I was angry – more with myself - feeling I should have done… SOMETHING…and wondering why I didn't see this coming, avoiding the admission that I did see it coming if only I had paid attention to the quiet inner voice that always guided me where I needed to be and that, once again, I chose to blow off. Over the weeks following Rose's death, the recurring thought of "Why didn't I call?" hammered away at me, twisting my insides, battering myself into a state of unparalleled frustration.

It's a neat trap for caregivers, thinking we can help everyone all the time, even though reality does its best to keep our inflated egos in check.

Providing myself some solace by thinking Rose was exactly where she wanted to be, reunited with Pete, it dawned on me that here was another reason Sally and I were guided into taking this rollercoaster ride from hell. Being enriched with our own cancer experience, and the support I was able to provide Rose and Abby, I started to realize we had the tools to help so many other people who were entering the cancer ring for the first time. I wasn't sure how, but I knew that giving back in some tangible way was on my horizon.

Specific death and dying subjects to address:

Notes:

Caregiver Tip #19

Don't shy away from conversations about money and finances.

The cost of medical care in the U.S. ...well, you probably know already. The financial condition of the patient and/or caregiver has to be examined, with an eye toward how treatment will be paid for without bankrupting anyone involved. This is another hard conversation which involves everything from how the bills will be paid to the aftercare needs of the patient. Will the patient be home or in assisted living? What's the cost of assisted living versus home healthcare? Who would be the better caregiver in the given situation? Will the whole family be involved in financial decisions concerning care? While these are practical questions, they are also emotional questions. Work to get everyone concerned on the same page, otherwise the door is left open for resentments and tension -- the last two things anyone needs.

There is a lot to consider depending on your particular situation; it's easy to get overwhelmed. Refer to the caregivers mantra: ASK FOR HELP, whether from family or professional financial guidance.

It helps to work with people who know what they are doing. On our very first MSK visit, after filling out the reams of paperwork, an intake specialist sat with us to review everything. Most of that is a blur, but one thing she said startled and comforted me simultaneously.

"You don't need to worry about dealing with insurance. We will take care of everything for you. You need to focus on treatment and healing."

I realized that the medical guidance we received was not the only reason to maintain our gratitude.

Once the lymphoma diagnosis was solidified, my boss insisted I look into the Family Medical Leave Act, or FMLA. The most important aspect of this program is a guarantee of employment, which has the benefit of keeping medical insurance in place. As with any government or insurance program, the paperwork is always the hardest part, but it was worth the effort.

Sally and I were relatively healthy and young. We fell into that bracket where we still were of working age and had full expectations of coming out of this journey whole with minimal financial impact. Walking the floors of the hospital, it was easy to feel gratitude for our situation. We weren't dealing with advanced age, dementia, Alzheimer's, possible long-term care, childhood cancers, a less than hopeful prognosis -- all of this adds additional layers of emotional stress and increases the possibility of financial complications.

Then it hit me like an 18-wheeler - what about the people who have NO insurance? How can they afford treatment? Some of the bills and medical statements had arrived at home, and total costs were now well into the high six-figure realm... and climbing.

So, how do you decide what the priorities are - paying the mortgage or paying for life-saving treatment? A recent Chicago Tribune article stated the issue in succinct terms:

"Sometimes treating cancer means going broke."

There is even an official name for this situation: **cancer-related financial toxicity.** And while patient advocate groups battle out drug prices with the government and big Pharma in hopes of keeping costs down, this holds little immediate comfort for the family whose eight-year-old daughter is battling leukemia or six-year-old son fights tumors on his spine.

ASK FOR HELP

Appendix C contains a list of possible financial resources. It is by no means exhaustive but offers places to start. If nothing else, this journey taught me that the more people I talked to, the better connected to what we needed appeared. One contact always leads to another.

Financial resources with whom to connect:

_____
_____
_____
_____
_____
_____
_____
_____
_____
_____
_____

Financial topics of conversation:

_____
_____
_____
_____
_____
_____
_____

Notes:

Caregiver Tip #20

Give yourself credit.
Learn to accept praise from others.

It may not seem like it, but caregiving takes courage - almost as much courage as it does being a patient. Others will recognize that in you and offer their admiration for your actions. Realize they are being sincere, and mentally give yourself a pat on the back. This is hard work - mentally and ofttimes physically. Friends and family understand the toll it takes and will want to recognize your efforts.

"You're a good man."

That phrase was spoken to me by more than one of my friends. My usual response was a non-committal shrug of the shoulders. I never believed what I did, or didn't do, was cause for this kind of appreciation. I mean, really. All I did was sit on the sidelines and watch the game unfold. Like a water-boy I would dash onto the field on occasion to supply some needed relief, but I couldn't see my contribution as much beyond that.

We had experienced ten rounds of chemo over a six-month period and were on the precipice of the stem-cell transplant process. The intensity increased but I still saw myself as little more than a bystander.

Stem cell harvest day had finally arrived. Sally was hooked up to a machine that looked like a cross between R2D2 and a hardware store paint mixer, complete with spinning dials, and humming innards; I kept waiting for droid beeps and pings, or at least a projected hologram of Princess Leia, "Help me Obi-wan Kenobi...."

I watched in awe as Sally's blood came out through one of her two port channels, slurped into the machine where it separated into white cells, red cells and plasma. Stem cells are collected from the white cells, and then all three are subjected to the machine's VitaMix setting to get recombined and transported back in Sal's body through her second port channel. Who thinks of this stuff? I had images of two people tinkering in their garage, a la Steve Jobs and Bill Gates, constructing this gizmo out of spare parts from a dishwasher and an ancient John Deere lawn tractor.

Sally's stem cell squigglies were tucked safely in the Sloan deep freeze. All that remained was getting mentally psyched for the whole experience. Thinking back on our first treatment visit in November, we were skeptical and fearful of everything the hospital threw at us. It was all unknown. With the stem cell transplant, we accepted all the advice and council provided to us by doctors, nurses and previous stem cell transplant patients. Our defensive shields had vanished.

"This is a different ballgame, huh?" I said. "Can you imagine having to do this first thing?"

"Never would have happened," Sally said. "It's easy now. I just give them my keys, and do whatever they tell me to do."

My Two-Step Caregiver Stem Cell Transplant Prep Guide
(highly recommended prep steps)

1. Take a sheet of fine sandpaper, anything rated 300 grit or higher will do, and begin a daily regimen of scraping the skin behind your ears right where it joins the skull. Start this at least two weeks in advance so that by the time the transplant begins, a tough, foot-bunion skin forms at the ear-head joint. Without this, the elastic straps on the surgical masks, that you will wear constantly, will flay that tender skin into raw ground chuck in a matter of hours.[1]

2. Surgical gloves. On average I went through about 5-7 pairs a day. Nurses go through about 40 – 50 pairs a day. The hospital graciously provided three sizes. For guys with big hands, don't even monkey around with small or medium. You will herniate the flexor tendon in your thumb and possibly crack any number of metacarpal or phalange bones while attempting to jam your hand into the smaller sizes. Even if you do succeed, your hand will permanently cramp with pain that makes carpel tunnel syndrome feel like a full body massage. Go straight for the large size.

[1] Again this is pre-COVID so your ears may already be tougher that beef jerky.

It is an odd feeling, knowing that the stem cell transplant process takes a relatively healthy person and makes them unbelievably sick. To me that's like taking a sledgehammer to the windshield of a car in order to fix a flat tire. The plan was to spend a week being blasted by yet another chemo cocktail taking all Sally's blood levels to zero, re-introducing her stem cells, after thawing, and then spend a couple weeks waiting for the blood levels to tick back up. One side effect was that all Sally's basic childhood inoculations, measles, chicken pox, etc., were wiped out during the chemo process, leaving her vulnerable for the better part of a year until her cells were strong enough to grab on to the new inoculations.

When we checked in, we were assigned a room on the western side of the building that is within spitting distance of the next building on the block. This was New York after all. Sunlight was blocked, views were nonexistent, and the atmosphere was generally dreary and depressing. This was not going to work. The process would be tough enough without being sequestered like Papillon in solitary confinement. Whether Sally felt this or not didn't matter as I was the one tasked with keeping her spirits high. We were going to need at least some form of daylight to get through all this.

I was comfortable advocating by this point and upon meeting Patrice, our first nurse on transplant floor, I said, "Any way we can switch rooms to the other side of the building? This is kind of depressing, and we haven't even started yet."

"I get it," she said with a smile. "These back rooms are not the cheeriest places in the world. Let me see what I can do."

Within three hours, not only were we moved to the eastern side, but seriously upgraded to the first-class section - a corner room with eastern and southern views. Walking into the brightly-lit room, a sense of peace and relief washed over me. It was only day one, but I knew deep down everything was going to be okay.

Sally smiled at me and said, "Thanks."

"For what?"

"Advocating for me. I don't know that I would have spoken up about the room. I just would have accepted it. But this is so much better."

I smiled. "Sure you would have. This was nothing." What I should have said was just a simple "You're welcome". My old tapes of wanting to minimize everything were playing. It was something small, but in the long run, made a huge difference.

Our star stem-cell nurse, Elisabetta, radiated a "this is the way this is going to go down so get used to the idea" attitude. I loved her because I knew she would kick Sally's ass when she needed it, especially when my words of cheer fell on deaf ears.

Additionally, Elisabetta facilitated the Big Event.

The question, "To Shave or Not to Shave," had been paramount on Sally's mind since the brain biopsy. Up until the stem cell treatment, only minor hair losses were experienced, enough to invest in a wig, but not enough to go for the full-on Kojak look. Sally knew going in that complete hair-loss was a feature of the stem-cell protocol; hair follicles were sacrificed along with most every other cell in her body.

Elisabetta wielded the shaver the day Sally decided it was time to go bald. Enough hair had fallen out that there was little shaving to do anyway. I thought she looked great without hair —and this is from the guy who pestered her incessantly to grow it long, long, long.

An infusion nurse made the brilliant observation that women felt their hair was the last controllable aspect of their body at a time when everything felt out of control. When there is little to hold onto, even the smallest things bring a sense of sanity to the chaos. Sally and I had spoken about her hair several times. I made the offer to shave my head too in a show of support and solidarity.[2]

It was easy to support Sally and the hair loss because I honestly did think it was a look she could get away with. Most women can. Most men, particularly white men, cannot. Comedian Bill Engvall said it best: "Fifty percent of bald white men look like serial killers." Indeed.

Three weeks to the day after checking in, Sally was discharged, the first stage of the stem cell process completed. Leaving the hospital was bittersweet, especially for Sally. While she would desperately miss her nurse crew, once outside. both us were flooded with a sense of triumph. Driving away from the hospital with the windows open and inhaling her first breath of fresh air in nearly a month, Sally said, "Oh, God, that feels good."

"You did it," I said as I headed north on First Avenue, past all the storefronts and neighborhoods that had become so familiar to me during the previous year. Flashes of memory tore through my mind, conversations with restaurant owners, smells of Christmas trees, long walks to the New York Public Library on York Avenue. As much as the nurses, doctors and staff of Sloan had been Sally's world during the past year, this section of the East Side had become mine. I knew I would miss it.

"We did it," she said, looking at me with a mixture of love and awe. "I could not have done this without you."

"Oh, I think you would have made it if I wasn't here. Someone else would have filled my shoes, either Kate or the kids."

Okay, so as a caregiver, I still needed to work on accepting compliments and seeing the importance of my contributions. If nothing else, becoming a caregiver was a non-stop learning process.

---

2 Yeah, I know. I have a lot less hair to lose. Ha friggin' ha.

Opportunities to give myself credit or better accept praise from others:

_____
_____
_____
_____
_____
_____
_____
_____
_____
_____
_____
_____

Situations where I say "No problem" or "Not a big deal":

_____
_____
_____
_____
_____
_____
_____

Notes:

Caregiver Tip # 21

I'm sure you've noticed that everything has changed. Go easy on yourself while you adjust to the new norm.

When a loved one has cancer, everyone and everything else in the world appears to be "normal." Feeling quarantined in your new world is not unusual. Social media only aggrivates the perception that everyone else is fine and having fun while you, most certainly, are not. What you percieve as "normal" through cancer-colored glasses is a tricky deception; your "normal" is what you make of it. Sure, your new normal is different from the normal you were used to. However once the panic and fear subside, the new normal is an opportunity to re-imagine the possibilities of life anew with additional dimensions, regardless of treatment outcomes.

**It will take some time to adjust.
Be patient.**

No one told me I'd be giving birth at age 58. Newborn babies come home from the hospital and can do little but eat, sleep and poop as they don't have the skills to do much else. In addition - new moms back me up here - their trips outside are carefully monitored until they are about a year old and that first big round of immunizations hits.

That's what went down once we got home, the only difference being skill level. Sal was down for the count, energy wise, for some time. She did little but eat, sleep and poop, and she was severely restricted from being out in public with lots of germ-infested people for a year until she received all the basic childhood inoculations.

My life resembled Ward and June Cleaver combined; cooking, cleaning, laundry, shopping, dealing with two bratty four-legged kids[1] and a full-time job where my team was hanging my likeness in effigy, setting fire to it on a daily basis for all the good I was doing.[2]

Thank God for caffeine. Sleep was for the weak.

The emotional and physical toll of this final stem cell stage cannot be underestimated, especially for the patient. Sally and I talked about the ups and downs, the good and the bad of the whole process and while agreeing the long-term benefits outweigh the short-term possibilities, one of the

---

[1] One of whom was a **** hair away from being kicked out the door if he pooped in the house one more time.

[2] I don't recall any specific Leave It to Beaver episode where Ward was hung in effigy at his office, but I could be mistaken.

tougher things to stomach was spending June and July in the hospital while watching all our Facebook peeps post pictures from their various summer vacations. Sally and I are beach people. After skipping our usual week at the beach in 2014, it never occurred to us that the summer of 2015 would also pass without a beach vacation; that once again we would not get to Pt. Pleasant Beach on a Thursday night to watch the fireworks, get some frozen yogurt and people watch on the Boardwalk. Maybe we subconsciously knew it wasn't going to happen, but seeing our friends social media pictures and posts as they frolicked in the waves with their kids, or attended baseball games or hung around theme parks, hit home and made us both long for a normal summer again. We missed it desperately.[3]

Somewhere along the line I mentioned these feelings in a whining social media post. Our friends Stephanie and Rob paid us a visit at home, post-transplant, and presented Sally with a decorative glass jar filled with sand and small shells that they had put together while vacationing at the beach. Since Sally couldn't bask in the sand, they brought the sand to Sally. Heartfelt creativity rules.

One month later, 16 August 2015, Sally got the word from our stem-cell guru, Dr. Sauter; she was cleared to drive. For the first time in almost a year, Sally climbed in the driver's seat of her red Matrix and ventured out on her own. Donning mask and gloves, and without the usual escorts of me or Aunt Kate or anyone else, she headed out into the world. A little bit of freedom from the confinement of the past year. I can only imagine how good that must have felt.

We went to the bank one day, Sally wearing surgical mask and gloves. I said upon entering, "I hope they don't think this is a stick-up." She imme-

---

[3] Actually, that last bit about the theme parks not so much. We could skip that without too much distress.

diately brought up her hands with mock finger-guns pointing at the people in the bank. Lucky we're not in jail.

Sally was a star patient but is far from being a star at having patience; her desire to push the boundaries to get back to normal was a daily struggle. I've never seen anyone so frustrated at not being able to go into the basement to do laundry; she couldn't afford the exposure to mold yet. If I were in her shoes, I'd see that as a bonus, but Sally saw it as a burden on me and you know those Libras -- always more worried about inconveniencing others.

The other pain with the stem-cell recovery was the Low Microbial Diet. Not being able to eat raw veggies was brutal for someone like Sally who could eat salads three meals a day. Everything she consumed had to be cooked to death. Sally was more the raw, crunchy, medium-rare herbivore. Eating out was mostly verboten as well. We were told even a turkey sub and Diet Coke from Wawa was going to have to wait until next year. Sally, naturally, had her own timetable -- a fact I had grudgingly come to grips with as a caregiver - and by the six-month mark, Dr.Sauter told her she could start eating again.

Picking the important battles is a learned caregiving skill, especially when I started at a point of total ignorance, with sufficient fear to insist on following every instruction to the letter. Early on Sally's inquiries of, "Do I have to do this?" were always met with a firm and intractable, "Yes." After a year of treatments and transplants, my stance had relaxed, but, unfortunately, was far from the depressurization that I needed, as I found out the hard way.

Areas where I need to practice patience:

_____
_____
_____
_____
_____
_____
_____
_____
_____
_____
_____

Things I can do to center myself:

_____
_____
_____
_____
_____
_____

Notes:

Caregiver Tip # 22

As treatment wanes, take the time to decompress. It's okay, and sometimes necessary, to seek outside help

You've been carrying a heavy load for awhile and while the urge is to get back to pre-cancer "normal" as quickly as possible, you can't unless you let go of the burden you've been hauling around. This doesn't happen overnight, and you may not be able to do it alone. Most female caregivers understand this -- it's the guys I'm mainly addressing here. There is no shame in getting outside help - whether it's a social worker, therapist, psychiatrist, priest, rabbi, doctor, custodian, traffic cop...whatever professional makes you comfortable. An impartial third party can be very helpful when unusual thoughts start swirling in your head and driving into bridge abutments starts to look like a viable alternative.

"No, I'm not going to calm down. This is bullshit. What you are doing is wrong." I was screaming into the phone, at my boss, getting off on my own self-righteousness. "This shit has been going on far too long. Morale sucks and neither you nor any of the managers give a fuck about it." My outward raving was no match for the inner screaming, every nerve in my body was on fire, and I felt my energy expanding like a water balloon ready to burst.

My boss replied, calmly, "I'm not going to continue this conversation. I will call you back in 15 minutes when you've calmed down." To her credit, she didn't give me a chance to respond. The connection broke.

Fat flakes of snow continued to fall, blanketing the earth outside my home-office window. My rage still lashed out inside me; throwing a chair though a window or tearing a phone book in half felt like a reasonable action to take.

Six months had crawled by since the stem cell transplant, Christmas was two weeks away. Since Thanksgiving, I'd been sleeping far too late, not finding the will to get my ass out of bed by ten, eleven and some days noon. I had a built-in alibi – there was always something medical that needed attention. Whether there actually was a medical need or not was immaterial. Cancer trumped any and all conference calls.

The manic rollercoaster of emotions remained in play through the holidays. My energy and desire for anything remained at an all-time low. Each day was a slog of repetition: work, caretaking, cleaning, dog-sitting, cooking, laundry. An early snowstorm didn't help; for me, winter was death, the last stage in the life cycle. My tolerance for dealing with life's cycles had disappeared, swallowed up in 18 months of cancer, hospitals, medications and dying friends. Personal hygiene took a back seat, if I showered every couple of days, it was a lot. Staying up at night until two or three in the morning was not uncommon, planted in front of the TV or playing games on my phone. Subconsciously, I knew if I went to sleep, that meant I had to get up and deal with another day and all the responsibility and work insanity that went with it. Staying awake kept reality temporarily at bay.

One of the consequences of a bizarre upbringing was the hours of therapy I spent trying to make sense of my childhood and what I carried into adulthood. One of the benefits of hours of therapy is recognizing the earmarks of depression. I had blown a fuse at something work-related and inconsequential. As my fifth grade teacher, Miss Gaines, threatened me one day when my grades had bottomed out, the thread I was hanging by had broken.

I needed help.

My professional of choice at this time was a counsellor/coach named Theresa who had previously steered me through some very rough seas, at a time when I was seriously considering starting life anew, and had forced me to look deep inside, getting at the core of my unexpressed anger. It's almost always about suppressed anger or sadness or both.

"So what's going on?" Theresa asked when we settled in, her office bathed in the warm yellow lamplight of a standard living room. In talking through my rocky emotions with a professional, I came to realize that I had never taken the time to decompress after the treatment rollercoaster ended. I foolishly kept putting off my own emotional "stand-down" and continued doing my thing, working in a high-stress environment, trying to keep the house running, and keeping an eye on Sally at all times. I was exhibiting most of the classic symptoms of caregiver burnout syndrome.[1]

I started paying attention to my emotional status, how I was feeling at any given moment, and if I felt trapped and about to burst, I pulled back, kept my mouth shut, and turned whatever was happening over to my higher power.[2] I started taking more breaks, more time for myself – even if it was just reading or taking a nap. I made mental notes to breathe, all the tension has a habit of constricting basic physiological systems. I found ways to laugh – never discount the value of watching an old Marx Brothers movie.

By late spring, my boss and I were able to talk about the screaming incident.

"I really appreciate the help you've been to me lately. It's obvious you've gone through some big changes. Unless you've been faking it," my boss said one day.

I didn't respond to that comment. I'm not sure "faking it" qualifies as accurate. The stress of the workplace had grown exponentially since my winter explosion, the entire team was feeling it, but I used my caregiver recovery tools to muddle through it all. But even those only go so far.

On June 15, 2016 I finally cracked and quit my job outright. No two weeks' notice, I just left. Not exactly the classiest move but if I had to face one more day at work, I would have keeled over at my desk[3] or jumped

---

1 See Appendix B for a symptom checklist. It's a good thing to keep handy.

2 This is my own personal spirituality. You can worship green, near-sighted polar bears if that's what works for you. See Caregiver Tip # 7

3 Well, by this time I didn't have a desk anymore, I had a two-by-four foot table in a small room with three other people, but that's a whole different issue.

off the roof. I walked out of the building and felt as if I finally let go of a knapsack overloaded with encyclopedias.[4]

After my departure from work, I spent four weeks doing – nothing. It took that long before I started feeling somewhat human again, and before I stopped sitting bolt upright in bed fearing that I wasn't doing something I should have been doing. It took a minute to realize that muscle memory was playing games in my head, that there was nothing that needed immediate attention.

As I write this, it's been close to seven years since I bolted from Corporate America. I started my own voiceover business, and while that in and of itself has its own set of stresses, it's a significantly better way to live than where I was. The gratitude I have for being able to pull this off is immeasurable. What you hold in your hands, whether in wood pulp, electronic or audio form, is the result of wanting to give something back for all the care and blessings we received. Even if it never sells a copy, the benefits of chronicling it all to my own mental state of being are incredible.

---

[4] For you younger readers, encyclopedias used to be 26 massive hardbound books that weighed a ton. Trust me, the metaphor works for us older types.

Decompression actions I need to take:

_____
_____
_____
_____
_____
_____
_____
_____
_____
_____
_____
_____

Taking care of myself means:

_____
_____
_____
_____
_____
_____
_____

Notes:

Post Script

November 2016
Thanks Giving

---

21 November. It was two years ago today that we first walked into our new second home, Memorial Sloan Kettering Cancer Center, Room 715A. Time flies. It hardly seems possible. I'm not sure we could add much more to our list of things to be Thankful for this year.

When we returned to the hospital for the re-introduction of Sally's childhood inoculations, we made our normal round of visitations tracking down all those who took such good care of both of us. It did our hearts well to see the faces -- Sandra, Liz, Elisabetta, Tonia, Kristyn, Fariel, Katie, Millie, Shirley -- and for all those who were not around, you are always in our hearts.

While on the transplant floor, we ran into Tonia who mentioned that she had one patient who was having a tough emotional time in that ugly transplant space where chemo has ended, but the blood counts had not started coming back.

"Well, let's go," Sally said reaching for a mask and a pair of the familiar blue latex gloves.

"Awesome," Tonia said, leading Sally to the woman's room.

Most heroic deeds are quietly overlooked. The doctors, nurses, staff and certainly the patients all perform small heroic deeds on a daily basis, deeds that are rarely trumpeted in the news or acknowledged with ticker-tape fanfare. But that's okay. We started seeing the impact sharing our journey had on those around us.

During my corporate tenure, Tasha was my long-distance work wife, as she was for just about everyone in the company. Her positive attitude made Betty White seem like Oscar the Grouch. We had an additional connection, both of us carried Central Pennsylvania roots.

Tasha was visiting New Jersey for a business meeting, which naturally meant an after work gathering of some sort was in order. Corporate America has its deep-seated issues, but the bonds of friendship that are formed there are unbreakable.

Sally joined us for the afterwork festivities where Tasha and many others were in attendance.

Most of the people there knew of Sally's journey and were beyond gracious in their admiration and support. We ate, drank and laughed with these caring people until it was time to leave. As we said our goodbyes, I saw Tasha and Sally hugging and tears were streaking Tasha's face.

"I love seeing you because you give me hope," Tasha said. Her mother was enduring a similar cancer battle.

I thought about that moment and all the others as I strolled around the hospital corridor, replaying the recent past in my mind: the fears, the sleepless nights spent in the halls or curled up on waiting area sofas, the miraculous people who were now a permanent part of our lives. But most importantly, a quiet triumph that I'd been able to be there, for the experience, the doctors, nurses and especially Sally. Not everyone has a happy ending when it comes to cancer; we were lucky in that regard. I felt a sense of pride that I'd been able to perform all the caregiver functions, not always with a smile on my face I'll grant you, but I felt richer for the experience. I had weatheredan aspect of this process and, like Sally was doing at that moment, I knew I had to share my knowledge with others who needed it.

Sally and Tonia reappeared, and I could see from their faces that Sally had been able to reassure the patient that everything was going to be okay and that Sally was living proof of light at the end of the tunnel, and reaching that light is a series of a thousand steps, taking each, in order...

ONE

STEP

AT

A

TIME.

Caregiver Warriors

"Acknowledgements" lacks the "oomph" required for all the people who guided and supported us through our journey and continue to do so, and for those who waited far too patiently for this book to be completed. For me, this listing, more than the entire rest of the book, proves how blessed we truly are. If I have omitted your name, it is 100% negligence on my part - please forgive me.

Medicos:

Dr. Igor Gavrilovic, Dr. Michael Sauter, Dr. Seth Josepher, Dr. Nirav Shah, Dr. Michael Ye, Dr. Stephen Maslin Dr. Louis Tsarouhas

The Nurse Universe:

Practitioners: Dr. Liz Kelliher, Dr. Millie Gordillo-Guffanti, Dr. Lorraine Anderson

The best damn crew on the planet:

Kristyn Senzino, Alexa Baldassano, Jasmine Carrasquillo, Farial Bachas, Sandra Turzulli, Elisabetta Todari, Shirley Hendrickson, Nick Hendrickson, Katie Fox, Veronica Brown, Yasminda Muse, Petal Ann Persaud, Miche Dee, Kaitlin Whalley-Montross, Colleen Walsh, Sade Roshida Davis, Eleni Kalandranis, Tracy Collins, David, Raymond, Glenn, Marco, Tonia

Our Never-Fail friends:

Rich and Jill Brugger
Tom and Jane DiGirolamo
Nancy and Fred Golden
Nancy and Jeff Wilson
Tracy and Matt Kervik
Greg and Linda Harwood
Stephanie and Rob Rubin
Randy Fisher
Rosie Singlewatch
Helen Menzie-Higgins
Donya McCoy
The Westfield Senior High School Class of 1974 (and 1975)

Early Readers:

Michelene K., Ann Fry, Anne Dubisson Andersen

The "We Never Stop Working - Can You Hear Me Now?" Crew

Dina Jacobs, Tina Braley, Alan Kopacz, Joanna Zeh, Marie Moore, Jessica Luberger, Lori Wlazlowski, Mark Reitemeyer, Ana Lima, Leigh Lachman, Gabby Diogo, Vern Shaute, Katrina Pelican, Natasha Tafelski-Jones, John Walker, Sue and Rick Marchisio, Cindy Nichols, Jim Alexander, Scott Morelock, Mike and Rhonda Shannon, John and Kara Elward.

The entire POS UAT team, especially Seleesha Matthews and Carrie Kaler, who shouldered most of my absentee burden.

The Fam

The entire Cooper/Howard/Adams/Burgess/Young/Mawhinney/Gilmore/Budzilya clan, but especially Kate and Beth who remained constant guardians of home and the four-legged critters.

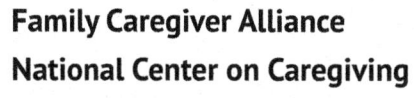

Appendix A: Caregiver Resources

Family Caregiver Alliance
National Center on Caregiving
785 Market Street, Suite 750
San Francisco, CA 94103
415-434-3388
800-445-8106
Website: www.caregiver.org
E-mail: info@caregiver.org
Family Care Navigator: www.caregiver.org/family-care-navigator

Memorial Sloan Kettering Cancer Center -mskcc.org
Today's Caregiver – www.caregiver.com
AARP – www.aarp.org

from CaringBridge.org

Appendix B: Signs of Caregiver Burnout

Physical symptoms:

- Rapid change in weight or appetite
- Body aches
- Migraines or persistent headaches
- Getting sick more often and for longer
- Exhaustion you can't shake, regardless of sleep

Emotional symptoms:

- Feeling hopeless, like your stress will never end
- Depression
- Anxiety/Panic attacks
- Feeling betrayed or alone
- Isolating yourself
- Low self-esteem, worthlessness

Appendix C: Financial Resources

This is by no means an exhaustive list. There are websites that specialize in lists of financial resources, such as **StupidCancer.org** and **ww5.komen.org** (that's not a typo - it really is ww5)

Cancer Financial Assistance Coalition (cfac) - CFAC is a coalition of organizations helping cancer patients manage their financial challenges.

https://www.cancerfac.org

Cancer Care dot Org- Sources of Financial Assistance

https://www.cancercare.org/publications/62-sources_of_financial_assistance

American Cancer Society - Programs and Resources to Help With Cancer-related Expenses

https://www.cancer.org

Susan G. Komen - How to Find Financial Assistance

https://ww5.komen.org/BreastCancer/FinancialResources.html

Patient Advocate Foundation - Patient Advocate Foundation (PAF) is a national 501 (c)(3) non-profit organization which provides case management services and financial aid to Americans with chronic, life threatening and debilitating illnesses.

https://www.patientadvocate.org/connect-with-services/financial-aid-funds/

The Pink Fund -The Pink Fund provides financial support to help meet basic needs, decrease stress levels and allow breast cancer patients in active treatment to focus on healing while improving survivorship outcomes.

https://www.pinkfund.org/get-help/

Strings For A Cure - StringsforaCURE® is an Erie, PA based 501(c)(3) non-profit charitable organization dedicated to providing education, comfort, financial assistance and emotional support directly to breast cancer patients.

http://www.stringsforacure.org/SFAC-Programs/

Family and Medical Leave Act (FMLA) - The FMLA entitles eligible employees of covered employers to take unpaid, job-protected leave for specified family and medical reasons with continuation of group health insurance coverage under the same terms and conditions as if the employee had not taken leave.

https://www.dol.gov/agencies/whd/fmla

Allyson Whitney Foundation - The Allyson Whitney Foundation primarily provides young adult cancer patients with 'Life Interrupted Grants™' to ease their financial burden, so that they can concentrate their energy on healing.

https://www.allysonwhitney.org/grants/

Cancer dot Net - the American Society of Clinical Oncology (ASCO) is the voice of the world's cancer physicians. ASCO's patient information website brings the expertise and resources of ASCO to people living with cancer and those who care for and care about them.

https://www.cancer.net/navigating-cancer-care/financial-considerations/financial-resources

Livestrong - An extensive list of financial resources. We ask survivors and caregivers what they need, we ask the system how it can be more person-centered, we ask innovators how we can bring impossible ideas to life.

https://www.livestrong.org/we-can-help/insurance-and-financial-assistance/health-care-assistance-for-uninsured

Bone Marrow & Cancer Foundation - The Bone Marrow & Cancer Foundation supports patients, their families and caregivers every step of the way during a cancer diagnosis or bone marrow, stem cell or cord blood transplant.

https://bonemarrow.org/support-and-financial-aid/financial-assistance

Bibliography

https://www.chicagotribune.com/lifestyles/ct-life-debt-from-cancer-20180520-story.html

AARP, National Alliance for Caregiving, "Caregiving in the US"; 2015

Gallup-Healthways. "Gallup-Healthways Well Being Index." 2011

About the Author

At one time or another, Jim Cooper has been a radio DJ, newspaper boy, worked retail in a department store paint section, a men's clothing shop and record store, been a commercial real estate broker, residential home builder, movie critic, IT programmer and project leader; owned his own IT consulting firm and home bakery business (not simultaneously), and currently owns Jim Cooper VO, narrating eLearning modules and audiobooks of all types. And that's just on Mondays. He is a music geek, still preferring vinyl to electronic forms of music, an avid reader and has recently jumped headfirst into the ancestry craze.

He has been blessed with a wife of 40+ years, two outstanding kids, three rambunctious granddaughters, and a never-ending string of insane rescue mutts.

His first book, *Twisted Ties*, a mystery novel, was published in 2014.

On your next vacation, visit Delaware.

Made in the USA
Columbia, SC
17 July 2025